CANCER ETIOLOGY, DIAGNOSIS AND TREATMENTS

GASTROINTESTINAL STROMAL TUMORS IN ADULTS AND CHILDREN

CANCER ETIOLOGY, DIAGNOSIS AND TREATMENTS

Additional books in this series can be found on Nova's website under the Series tab.

Additional e-books in this series can be found on Nova's website under the e-book tab.

CANCER ETIOLOGY, DIAGNOSIS AND TREATMENTS

GASTROINTESTINAL STROMAL TUMORS IN ADULTS AND CHILDREN

ATIF A. AHMED
EDITOR

New York

Library of Congress Cataloging-in-Publication Data

ISBN: 978-1-63483-679-1

Library of Congress Control Number: 2015948677

Published by Nova Science Publishers, Inc. † New York

CONTENTS

FORWARD

Gastrointestinal stromal tumor (GIST) is a great example of how science can impact outcomes in cancer patients. As a malignancy, GIST was not recognized as its own disease until 1983 when pathologists M.T. Mazur and H.B. Clark first coined the neutral term "Gastric Stromal Tumor" to encompass gastrointestinal non-epithelial neoplasms that lacked the immuno-histochemical features of Schwann cells and did not have the ultrastructural characteristics of smooth muscle cells. At the molecular level, GIST has fewer changes in its genome than most other solid cancers. Thus, the discovery in 1998 that GIST contained mutations in the *c-KIT* gene (the normal cellular homologue of the Hardy Zuckerman 4 feline sarcoma viral oncogene) and later the *PDGFRA* gene was a breakthrough for advancing the biology and treatment of GIST. However, these discoveries were just the beginning of unraveling the complexity of this disease; more accurately these diseases with both known and unknown causative genetic abnormalities. Introduction of tyrosine kinase inhibitors such as imatinib mesylate (also known as Gleevec™), an oral 2-phenylaminopyrimidine derivative that acts as a selective inhibitor against several receptor tyrosine kinases including KIT, PDGFRA, and BCR-ABL, significantly improved the outcomes for most GIST patients, who previously faced very poor prognosis. Clinicians at the bedside of their patients have seen the impact of imatinib and other drugs and have also had to face the challenges of what to do when a novel, promising therapy fails. Unfortunately, about half of the metastatic GIST patients treated with imatinib will have their tumor start to grow again within 2 years. Despite the dramatic progress in GIST treatment brought by imatinib, the development of primary and secondary resistance is a substantial obstacle that continues to mandate exploring other therapy alternatives, such as sutent and regorafenib. The study of GIST, both in the clinic and at the bench, has provided an odyssey of hope and despair for patients with this often fatal disease. Atif Ahmed's "Gastrointestinal Stromal Tumors in Adults and Children," assembles the view of several experts in the field to succinctly assess past and recent advancements in the diagnosis and treatment of patients with GIST. Clinicians, clinical scientists, and basic investigators, both old and new to the field, will undoubtedly learn more about GIST by reading this book and will better understand some of the challenges that lie ahead that must be overcome if we hope to further impact the lives of patients who are looking for answers and cures.

Andrew K. Godwin, PhD
Chancellors Distinguished Chair in Biomedical Sciences Endowed Professor
Professor, Department of Pathology & Laboratory Medicine,
University of Kansas Medical Center
Director, Molecular Oncology, University of Kansas Medical Center
Deputy Director, University of Kansas Cancer Center
Kansas Bioscience Authority Eminent Scholar

PREFACE

Gastrointestinal stromal tumors (GIST) are unique genetically-defined mesenchymal neoplasms affecting the gastrointestinal tract. These tumors account for approximately 1% - 3% of all malignant gastrointestinal tumors with an estimated incidence of approximately 5,000 new cases in the United States per year and an annual worldwide incidence ranging from 11 to 14.5 per million population. Tumors in adults and children have evolved as distinct genetic entities that exhibit significant differences in presentation, diagnosis and biologic behavior.

GIST has been and still is the subject of fervent research that has resulted in change of nomenclature, classification, diagnosis and treatment over the last 20 years. A Medline search for the term "gastrointestinal stromal tumor" has resulted in more than 5000 publications in the last decade with a peak of >600 in the last year. Significant advances in translational research and management have been made and documented through more than 200 clinical trials. The management of this disease and its associated morbidity frequently result in considerable hospital and other health costs that include both direct and indirect costs. Additional costs are incurred through pharmacy, monitoring of patients during and after initial treatment and treatment of relapse.

This book intends to provide a deep insight into the current research on the subject and summarizes all the important relevant basic and clinical data. It is intended for researchers, clinicians, radiologists, surgeons, pathologists and all those who are involved in the care of patients with this tumor. Chapters are authored by prominent researchers and clinicians of different specialties from the United States and across the globe.

Chapter 1 serves as an introductory chapter into the diagnosis, pathophysiology, treatment and prognosis of GIST. GIST arise most commonly as sporadic tumors in adults, and rare cases may be familial and/or develop in childhood. Clinical manifestations vary, however gastro-intestinal bleeding is the most common presentation. Treatment of GIST requires multidisciplinary care. Surgery is required for definitive management of early stage GIST and may be useful in advanced disease. The medical management of this disease has been revolutionized by the discovery of imatinib mesylate and other tyrosine kinase inhibitors (TKI) and their proven role in the management of late stage and high risk early stage tumors.

Chapter 2 summarizes a decade-history in the research of GIST and the discovery of mutations in the genes of two receptor tyrosine kinases, namely normal cellular homologue of the Hardy Zuckerman 4 feline sarcoma viral (v-Kit) oncogene (c-*KIT*) and platelet-derived growth factor receptor A (*PDGFRA*). These gain-of-function mutations are oncogenic drivers for GIST development and progression and are the target of imatinib, which has a strong and specific inhibitory action on relevant receptor tyrosine kinases aberrant signaling. The identification of mutations in these driver genes and the recently identified genetic signatures play important role in GIST diagnosis, staging, therapy, management and prognosis. Molecular analysis is now an inseparable part of the current personalized approach to clinical management of GIST patients.

Chapter 3 looks in depth into the various imaging studies used in the clinical management of primary and metastatic GIST. Imaging studies are useful in determining the exact location and size of the tumor, attenuation, aggressiveness of the tumor and metastatic deposits. Metastasis at presentation is seen in more than 50% of cases, most commonly to the liver followed by peritoneum. Computed tomography (CT) is the gold standard modality in the initial diagnosis and staging of GIST. Positron emission tomography combined with CT is the investigation of choice for assessment of response by virtue of its unique dynamic functional characteristics.

Chapter 4 discusses surgical resection as the principal treatment for GIST. Several factors, including tumor stage (i.e., localized, metastatic or multifocal disease), size, location, involvement of adjacent organs, proximity to critical structures, and presenting symptoms/signs are important to consider in operative decision-making. The primary goal of surgical resection is to achieve total gross resection of disease with microscopically negative margins while maintaining an intact pseudocapsule, sparing adjacent organs uninvolved by tumor, and only resecting clinically positive lymph nodes. The patient's overall health status should be considered in these decisions and a multidisciplinary approach is warranted in the care of all GIST patients. The use of neoadjvuant and adjuvant TKI therapies should also be contemplated in appropriately selected patients that may benefit in terms of a more limited resection, increasing the likelihood of resecting all gross disease, or decreasing the risk of recurrence.

Chapter 5 discusses the pathologic diagnosis of GIST with histology, cytology and immunohistochemistry. Regardless of patient's age and tumor location, GIST tumors are characterized by similar gross and microscopic details. The diagnosis is suspected by identifying the spindle cell, epithelioid or mixed stromal morphology and confirmed by immunohistochmical staining with CD117, CD34 and/or DOG1. Molecular diagnostic tests for *KIT* and *PDGFR* mutations are becoming increasingly available to confirm the diagnosis and aid in patient's management. Prognostic markers should be identified during pathologic examination and molecular testing.

In Chapter 6, the authors describe GIST in young children as a unique entity with striking differences from those in adults. Most GIST in young children are wild type for *KIT* and *PDGFRA* oncogenes and arise by different mechanisms. They are frequently associated with tumor-specific loss of the succinate dehydrogenase (SDH) complex function, which can be detected by immunohistochemical loss of expression or mutational testing, and are thus designated SDH-deficient GIST. SDH-deficient GIST occur in Carney-Stratakis syndrome and Carney Triad, exhibit different biologic behavior and do not follow the same prognostic parameters, like in adults. Tyrosine kinase inhibitors are not effective in treating SDH-deficient GIST. Knowledge of these biologic and behavioral differences is important in the management of young children with GIST.

In Chapter 7, the authors review the lengthy management of GIST with tyrosine kinase inhibitors. Surgery followed by adjuvant treatment with imatinib for three years is the standard of care in high risk tumors. Neoadjuvant imatinib is increasingly being used for locally advanced unresectable tumors at presentation. For patients with advanced GIST, the Food and Drug Administration has approved three drugs – imatinib, sunitinib and regorafenib. The authors also discuss the cost-effectiveness and relevance to the use of these drugs in India, as an example of a developing country. Although imatinib has quite a few generic versions available for use in India, there are currently no generic drugs available for sunitinib and regorafenib.

The last two chapters discuss current ongoing research and future directions in the management of this tumor. Patients could benefit from future research focusing on the identification of novel biomarkers with diagnostic and therapeutical value, discovery of novel genes and mutations associated with initiation and progression of the disease, novel therapeutics discoveries and advances in GIST therapy, and implementation of novel methods for disease detection and therapy monitoring. The identification of new molecules, beyond TKI is highly needed. Chapter 9 also highlights the state of the art of GIST management, with particular focus on treatment-resistant patients and wild-type GIST.

Atif A. Ahmed, MD
Staff Pathologist and Associate Professor,
University of Missouri
Department of Pathology and Laboratory Medicine,
Children's Mercy Hospital and Clinics,
2401 Gillham Road, Kansas City, MO 64108, US
Email: aahmed@cmh.edu

July 2015

In: Gastrointestinal Stromal Tumors in Adults ... ISBN: 978-1-63483-679-1
Editor: Atif A. Ahmed

Chapter 1

INTRODUCTION TO GIST: EPIDEMIOLOGY, CLINICAL FEATURES AND DIAGNOSTIC WORK-UP

Samuel Harris, Charlotte Benson and Robin L. Jones [*]
Sarcoma Unit, Royal Marsden Hospital
Fulham Road, London, UK

ABSTRACT

Gastrointestinal stromal tumours (GIST) are rare mesenchymal tumours of the GI tract, occurring most commonly in the stomach. The recognition of the *KIT* gene, the role it has in the development of GIST and the ability to treat the disease with tyrosine kinase inhibitors have revolutionised the diagnosis, treatment and prognosis of GIST. GISTs arise most commonly as sporadic tumours in adults, however rare cases may be familial and/or develop in childhood. Somatic mutations of the *KIT* gene are responsible for approximately 80% of cases, with *PDGFR* mutations and SDH deficiency responsible for the majority of other cases. Clinical manifestations vary; however, gastro-intestinal bleeding is the most common presentation. Treatment of GIST requires multidisciplinary care. Surgery is required for definitive management of early stage GIST and may be useful in advanced disease. Medical management with

[*] Correspondence: Robin L Jones, MD. Sarcoma Unit, Royal Marsden Hospital, Fulham Road, London, SW3 6JJ. Telephone: 0207 808 2137; Fax: 0207 808 2113; Email: rjones@seattlecca.org; Robin.jones@rmh.nhs.uk.

imatinib or other tyrosine kinase inhibitors has a proven role in the management of late stage disease and as adjuvant therapy in high risk early stage tumours.

Epidemiology

Gastrointestinal Stromal Tumours (GISTs) are rare malignancies, accounting for less than 1% of all gastrointestinal tumours, however, they are the most common mesenchymal tumours of the gastrointestinal tract [1].

GIST is a relatively new diagnosis, being first described in 1983 and was under diagnosed until the early 2000's when the activating mutations in *KIT* and *PDGFRA* were discovered [2]. Previously they were classified variously as leiomyomas, leiomyosarcomas, leiomyoblastomas and other rare entities [3].

Using modern diagnostic criteria the incidence has been estimated at between 7-15 cases per million people. Large population based studies that allowed histopathological confirmation from Sweden, Netherlands and Iceland found the incidence to be 14.5, 12.7 and 11 case per million respectively [4-6]. A SEER database analysis from USA in 2011 estimated the incidence to be 7.8 per million people. This had increased from 5.5 per million in the same database over a ten year period, reflecting, most likely, better diagnosis rather than a true increasing incidence [7].

It is, however, difficult to know the true incidence of GISTs. Many GISTS are small, indolent and may never be diagnosed or reported to registries [3]. It has been estimated that only 20-35% of GISTs are overtly malignant. Recent studies have highlighted the possibility of a higher incidence of small GISTs. A study looking at autopsy specimens from patients with gastric cancer found incidental microscopic GISTs (all less than 0.5 cm) in 35 out of 100 patients. This suggests that small GISTs are more common than previously recognized, and it is likely that many never develop into larger tumours, or do so very slowly [8].

GISTs are most common in middle aged and older patients. The mean age of diagnosis of GISTs is approximately 65 years of age with a peak incidence in the 70-79 year old [3, 7]. GISTs are rare under the age of thirty, although paediatric and young adult GISTs do occur, accounting for approximately 0.5-2.7% of GISTs [9]. GISTs may be more common in men, the SEER database analysis found GISTs to be 36% more common in men with a Rate Ratio (RR) of 1.35, a finding replicated in a systematic review of 4534 patients [7, 10].

However, some larger series have found no difference between the sexes [4, 11]. Paediatric and wild type GISTs are more frequent in women [9, 12]. The SEER analysis also suggested increased rates amongst Hispanic (RR 1.23), black (RR 2.07) and Asian (RR 1.5) populations, as compared to white populations [7].

The vast majority of GISTs are sporadic, however, a number of familial causes have been described - responsible for less than 5% of cases [13]. Germline mutations in *KIT*, *PDGRFA*, *NF1* and *SDH* have all been associated with GIST. Families with inherited *KIT* mutations tend to have variable clinical pictures that often include skin hyperpigmentation, urticaria pigmentosa, and dysphagia. The majority of the mutations described were exon 11, although exon 13 and 17 mutations have also been described [14]. *PDGFRA* mutations have been described in a few families and are often associated with large hands. Neurofibromatosis type 1 (NF1) is a relatively common autosomal dominant genetic disorder associated with café au lait spots, dermal neurofibromas, freckling and ocular harmartomas. It is caused by mutations in the *NF1* gene that encodes the neurofibromin protein responsible for GTPase activation. Patients with NF1 have a higher risk of gastrointestinal malignancies of which GIST are thought to account for over 30% [15]. GISTs associated with NF1 are generally not associated with *KIT* or *PDGFRA* mutations and may have better prognosis than other GISTs [16]. The Carney-Stratakis Syndrome (CSS) is an autosomal dominant familial disorder in which patients develop GISTs and paragangliomas, although there is incomplete penetrance [17]. It was originally described as being caused by mutations in genes for subunits B, C or D of Succinate Dehydrogenase (*SDH*) [18]. More recently germline mutations in the *SDH* subunit A have been reported [19]. *SDH* is a mitochondrial enzyme that is part of both the citric acid cycle and electron transport chain. It may also have a tumour suppressor function [14, 20].

GISTs are rare in the paediatric population, accounting for 0.5-2.7% of all GISTs [9]. The annual incidence may be as low as 2 cases per 100 million children [21]. However those that do occur have distinct epidemiological, pathological and clinical features. Paediatric GISTs tend to occur in females, most commonly with chronic GI bleeding. Multifocal tumours are common, as are lymph node metastases. The clinical behaviour of paediatric GISTs, although they are often metastatic, tends to be more indolent. GIST related mortality has been reported as less than 10% with median survival of 16 years in one series [22]. It is unusual for a paediatric GIST to harbour the classic activiating *KIT* or *PDGFRA* mutations. Conversely, paediatric GISTS are often syndromic, particularly Carney Triad and Carney-Stratakis Syndrome. Carney Triad is defined as the presence of pulmonary chondroma, GIST and paraganglioma, although may be suspected when any 2 of the three diagnoses are present. Carney Triad is thought to be sporadic as distinct from Carney Stratakis Syndrome described above [18].

HISTORY OF GIST

The diagnosis of GIST is a relatively new diagnosis. Traditionally GISTs were classified as smooth muscle neoplasms, based on morphology. As such they were usually classified as leiomyoma, leiomyosarcomas, leiomyoblastomas and other rare diseases. During the 1960's and 1970's it became apparent from electron microscopic studies that many did not have smooth muscle differentiation [23]. In 1983 the term "Gastrointestinal Stromal Tumour" was coined by Mazur and Clark in recognition that these neoplasms were a distinct entity [24]. However, the diagnosis was rarely made until around 2000. In 1998, Hirota and colleagues identified a gain of function mutation in the *cKIT* gene, which was present in most GISTs [25]. Subsequently the development of the immunohistochemistrical marker CD117 which corresponded to *KIT*, was found to be nearly universally expressed in GISTs, allowed easier recognition and diagnosis of this disease [26]. In 2001, imatinib an oral tyrosine kinase inhibitor against *KIT*, was demonstrated to be very active in GIST and this prompted a proliferation of interest and research into GIST leading into the modern era of successful therapy and clinical trial recruitment [27].

PATHOLOGY

The histological appearance of GISTs can be varied, however three main morphological appearances have been described – spindle cell (70%), epithelioid type (20%) and mixed 10% [28]. Spindle cell GISTs have relatively uniform cells arranged in fascicles. They have an overall basophilic appearance due to high nuclear density and scant cytoplasm. Nuclear palisading and juxtanuclear cytoplasmic vacuoles are often seen. Epithelioid GISTs have round to polygonal cells with variably basophilic cytoplasm and round nuclei. Mixed GISTs may have abrupt transitions between the two appearances or more complex intermingling [28, 29]. Although there is conflicting data, the different histological appearances do not seem to have prognostic influence [28, 30, 31].

Although the histological features can be suggestive of the diagnosis of GIST, they are not specific, and the final diagnosis relies upon immuno-histochemical (IHC) markers. The most important immunohistochemical markers for GIST are CD117 and DOG1. CD117 is the protein expressed by the *KIT* gene, and is positive in 90-95% of cases of GISTs, although may be negative in *PDGFRA* related GISTs. CD117 does not necessarily equate to *KIT* mutation, as the *KIT* gene may be overactive resulting in CD117 expression in non-*KIT* mutated GISTs especially paediatric or wild-type GISTs. CD117 may also be positive in non-GIST tumours including melanoma and Kaposi's sarcoma. DOG1 is a more recently discovered imunohistochemical marker that has both excellent sensitivity and specificity for GIST. It is positive in 96-99% of GISTs, including PDGFA related GISTs and has a specificity of >99% for GIST. As such, DOG1 and CD117 have become the IHC markers of choice for the diagnosis of GIST. Another IHC marker that may be useful is CD34, which is positive in up to 81% of cases, although it has much lower specificity [26, 29].

MUTATION STATUS AND MOLECULAR SUBTYPES

GISTs are commonly classified in relation to the underlying genetic mutation that can be identified. *KIT, PDGFRA*, *SDH* deficient, *BRAF* are the mutations that have been identified to date, and account for nearly 90% of all GISTs.

KIT Mutations

KIT mutated GISTs are the most common of all GISTs, accounting for up to 80% of all cases. The *KIT* gene enocodes a transmembrane receptor, that becomes constitutively activated in the presence of a *KIT* mutation. This leads to increased downstream signalling that drives cellular proliferation and survival. *KIT* mutated GISTs are generally sensitive to imatinib. Exon 11 (which codes the intracellular juxtamembrane domain of the protein) mutations are the most common, accounting for approximately 70% of GIST *KIT* mutations. These mutations are particularly sensitive to inhibition with imatinib – an oral tyrosine kinase inhibitor that targets the KIT protein. Exon 9 (extracellular domain) making up 5-20%, are less sensitive to imatinib. Exon 13 (approximately 1-4%) and Exon 17 (approximately 1%) mutations are much less common [3, 32].

PDGFRA Mutations

Platelet Derived Growth Factors Receptor Alpha mutations are seen in between 5-10% of all GISTs. Mutation of this gene causes constituent activation and increased downstream signalling of cellular processes leading to tumour growth. In a similar fashion to *KIT*, different exons are responsible for different portions of the protein. Although *PDGFRA* mutated GISTs may respond to imatinib, particular *PDGFRA* mutations have been found to be highly resistant, particularly the *PDGFRA D842V* mutation [32].

BRAF Mutations

BRAF mutations are rare, accounting for less than 1% of all GISTs. However, in population of GISTs confirmed to be *PDGFRA/KIT* negative, they account for about 10%. *BRAF* mutation and activation lead to increased activity in the MAPK pathway. Although little is known about these tumours, they may respond to *BRAF* inhibitors [33].

SDH Deficiency

Succiante Dehydrogenase (SDH) is a four protein complex (Subunits A, B, C and D) that acts in the mitochondria in the interphase between the electron transport chain and tricarboxylic acid cycle. Loss of any of the SDH subunits lead to SDH deficiency and has been associated with tumourigenesis. SDH deficiency is commonly seen in paediatric GIST, and maybe sporadic or germline or, as seen with Carney Stratakis Syndrome. SDH deficient GISTs seem to be isolated to Gastric GISTs, and account for approximately 7.5% of all gastric GISTS [34].

Wild Type GIST

Wild type GIST is a changing definition, and might better be described as GISTs with no identified gain of function mutation. This is a small group responsible for a minority of cases of GIST.

Prognostic Factors

The risk of recurrence after surgery for GIST is highly variable and depends on a number of risk factors. Based on a number of large retrospective studies; tumour size, mitotic rate and anatomical site have all been validated as independent risk factors for relapse after resection [31, 35-37]. Increasing tumour size is associated with increasing risk of relapse, with tumours <2 cm rarely or never developing metastases. The risk increases with increasing size above 2 cm, 5 cm and 10 cm. Increasing mitotic rate is also of prognostic importance, with <=5 mitotic figures per 50 high power fields associated with better prognosis than >5/50 HPF [28]. Small Bowel and rectal GISTs have higher risks of relapse than gastric GISTs [36]. Tumour rupture also seems to be a risk for recurrence, although less validated than the other known risk factors, with nearly 100% recurrence seen after tumour rupture reported in one series [38].

More recently it has been shown that the underlying mutation also has prognostic implications. In a multivariate analysis of 1505 GISTs, found that the presence of a *KIT* mutation was associated with increased recurrence risk compared to *PDGFRA* and WT GIST. However, this was less important than the standard risk factors discussed above. There was no significant difference between Exon 9, 11, 13 and 17 *KIT* mutations in the multivariate analysis for recurrence. However there were individual mutations that predicated better or worse outcomes. For example a duplication mutation in *KIT* exon 11 was associated with significantly lower risk of recurrence and *KIT* exon 9 mutation leading to Ala502_Tyr503 duplication was a high risk mutation. Despite this, the traditional risk factors, were more accurate in predicting recurrence, for example a <2 cm GIST will have a very low risk of recurrence regardless of the underlying mutation [39].

Based on these known risk factors, there has been a number of different risk stratification systems developed for predicting recurrence. These generally group recurrence risk into very low, low moderate and high risk groups [28, 36, 40, 41]. These risk stratification tables or nomograms are useful in helping to decide who should receive adjuvant therapy, which is generally recommended to patients with high risk of relapse [42]. One of the more common risk stratification systems is provided in Table 1.

Table 1 [36]. Risk Stratification of Primary GIST by Mitotic Index, Size, and Site

Tumor Parameters			Risk of Progressive Disease (%)			
Group	Size	Mitotic rate	Gastric	Jejunal/Ileum	Duodenal	Rectum
1	≤ 2 cm	≤ 5 per 50 hpf	None (0%)	None (0%)	None (0%)	None (0%)
2	>2 ≤ 5 cm		Very low (1.9%)	Low (4.3%)	Low (8.3%)	Low (8.5%)
3a	> 5 ≤ 10 cm		Low (3.6%)	Moderate (24%)	High (34%) ‡	High† (57%) ‡
3b	> 10 cm		Moderate (12%)	High (52%)		
4	≤ 2 cm	> 5 per 50 hpf	None†	High† (50%)	§	High (54%)
5	> 2 cm ≤ 5 cm		Moderate (16%)	High (73%)	High (50%)	High (52%)
6a	> 5 cm ≤ 10 cm		High (55%)	High (85%)	High (86%)‡	High (71%)‡
6b	> 10 cm		High (86%)	High (90%)		

† denotes tumor categories with very few cases.

‡ Groups 3a and 3b, 6a and 6b are combined in duodenal and rectal GISTs because of small number of cases.

§ No tumors of such category were included in the study.

Clinical Features

GISTs may arise from any location along the gastrointestinal tract. The stomach is the most common accounting for 40-60% of GISTs. Jejunal and ileal GISTs are the next most common, comprising 25-30% of all GISTS. Less frequent are colorectal (5-15%), duodenal (5%) and oeseophageal (<1%) GISTs. Very rarely, GISTs may arise from the mesentery, omentum or retroperitoneum and are referred to as extragastrointestinal stromal tumours [3, 43]. GISTs, especially paediatric, may be multifocal in nature [22].

Metastases from GIST are nearly always intra-abdominal. The liver, peritoneum and omentum are the most common locations for metastases. Pulmonary, bone and brain metastases are very rare, as are lymph node metastases [34]. However, paediatric GISTs are more likely to develop nodal metasatases [22].

GI bleeding, an abdominal mass, and abdominal pain are the most common forms of presentation for GIST. Early satiety, bloating, jaundice, dysphagia, fever and fatigue are other common presenting symptoms. Nearly 2/3 of patients have overt or occult GI bleeding at the time of diagnosis. Rarely perforation or obstruction may occur. A small proportion of GISTs are diagnosed incidentally from CT imaging or gastroscopy arranged for other reasons [10].

Approximately 10-25% of patients present with metastatic disease. Patients with metastatic disease may often have bulky disease prior to developing symptoms. Common symptoms of metastatic disease are bloating, abdominal distension, nausea, anorexia, weight loss and fatigue [3, 27].

INVESTIGATIONS

CT or PET/CT are the most useful imaging modalities for diagnosis and staging. GISTs appear, typically, on CT to be a solid mass with IV contrast enhancement. GISTs may appear exophytic or endopyhtic, sometime with dual components, the so called dumb-bell lesion. Larger lesions may have necrosis. GISTs are usually intensely FDG avid on PET/CT.

Endoscopic Ultrasound (EUS) is recommended for the investigation of gastric and upper small bowel GISTs. EUS allows guided fine needle aspiration which is highly sensitive and specific for diagnosing GIST [43]. Ultrasonographic evaluation of the lesion also allows characterization and can be very helpful in distinguishing benign from malignant lesions. Malignant features seen on EUS include: larger tumour size, irregular extra-luminal border, heterogeneity, echogenic foci and cystic spaces [44].

Biopsy prior to surgery is not always required, especially with lesions that are easily resectable and characteristic for GIST on imaging. However, for patients requiring neoadjuvant treatment or if there is diagnostic uncertainty, biopsies are recommended. If possible, fine needle aspiration with EUS is preferred over radiological guided percutaneous biopsy, because of the potential risk of tumour seeding, although percutaneous biopsy can be safe if performed in expert centres [45-47].

Some locally advanced tumours may benefit from pre-operative therapy with imatinib. Decisions regarding the use of pre-operative therapy should be made within the context of an experienced multi-disciplinary team.

TREATMENT

Optimal treatment of GIST requires specialist care as part of a multidisciplinary team. Surgery is the mainstay for treatment of localised disease and should be performed by surgeons skilled in the resection of GISTs. Resection en-bloc is required in order to obtain negative margins and to minimise the risk of tumour rupture and dissemination of micro-metastatic disease. Extensive loco-regional dissection is not required beyond what is required for negative margins as GISTs rarely metastasize to lymph nodes [3]. Although medical management is the cornerstone of treatment of advanced disease, surgery may also play a role for certain indications – although no prospective data exists. Based on a number of retrospective case series, in patients with oligo-metastatic disease, complete resection of the metastatic deposits may improve progression-free survival (PFS). Likewise resection of a focally progressing lesion in the setting of otherwise responsive disease on medical therapy may also improve outcomes. Continuation of medical therapy is required as the cessation of medical therapy post resection of metastases has been associated with substantially shorter relapse times [48, 49]. An alternative to surgery in patients with limited hepatic metastasis is radio-frequency ablation [50].

The medical treatment of GISTs has been revolutionised by developments in understanding of the biology and pathogenesis of GIST. Prior to the recognition of the importance of the *KIT* gene in GIST and the ability to target this, treatment for advanced disease was limited. Treatment was often given with doxorubicin or ifosfamide, however, response rates were extremely low, and primary resistance rates high and as such GISTs were considered chemotherapy resistant [51, 52]. The development of imatinib to target KIT revolutionised the medical treatment and led to substantial improvements in both short and long term survival [1]. Subsequent developments have led to effective second and third line treatments with sunitinib and regorafenib having shown benefit [53, 54]. Adjuvant therapy with imatinib for patients at high risk of progression has also been shown to improve survival [42]. The medical management of GIST is discussed at length in subsequent chapters.

Conclusion

GISTs are rare malignancies of the gastrointestinal tract. Understanding of the molecular biology of GISTs has driven the understanding and led to better diagnosis and classification of these tumours. Mutations in *KIT* gene are responsible for the vast majority of GISTs with *PDGRA*, *SDH* and *BRAF* mutations responsible for a small number. GISTs most commonly occur in older patients. Rarely, GISTs can occur in paediatric populations. Diagnosis is usually made with CT or PET/CT and endoscopic biopsy. Tumour size, location and mitotic rate are the most important prognostic factors in predicting recurrence. The use of Imatinib and other tyrosine kinase inhibitors have revolutionized the medical treatment of GIST.

References

[1] Judson I, Demetri G. Advances in the treatment of gastrointestinal stromal tumours. *Ann Oncol* 2007; 18(Suppl 10):x20–4.

[2] Nishida T, Hirota S. Biological and clinical review of stromal tumors in the gastrointestinal tract. *Histol Histopathol* 2000; 15(4):1293-301.

[3] Joensuu H. Gastrointestinal stromal tumor (GIST). *Ann Oncol* 2006; 17(suppl 10):x280–6.

[4] Nilsson B, Bümming P, Meis-Kindblom JM, et al. Gastrointestinal stromal tumors: The incidence, prevalence, clinical course, and prognostication in the preimatinib mesylate era-a population based study in western Sweden. *Cancer* 2005; 103(4):821–9.

[5] Goettsch WG, Bos SD, Breekveldt-Postma N, Casparie M, Herings RM, Hogendoorn PC. Incidence of gastrointestinal stromal tumours is underestimated: results of a nation-wide study. *Eur J Cancer* 2005; 41(18):2868–72.

[6] Tryggvason G, Gíslason HG, Magnússon MK, Jónasson JG. Gastrointestinal stromal tumors in Iceland, 1990-2003: The Icelandic GIST study, a population-based incidence and pathologic risk stratification study. *Int J Cancer* 2005; 117(2):289–93.

[7] Ma GL, Murphy JD, Martinez ME, Sicklick JK. Epidemiology of Gastrointestinal stromal tumors in the era of histology codes: Results of a population-based study. *Cancer Epidemiol Biomarkers Prev* 2015; 24(1):298–302.

[8] Kawanowa K, Sakuma Y, Sakurai S, et al. High incidence of microscopic gastrointestinal stromal tumors in the stomach. *Hum Pathol* 2006; 37(12):1527–35.

[9] Benesch M, Wardelmann E, Ferrari A, Brennan B, Verschuur A. Gastrointestinal stromal tumors (GIST) in children and adolescents: A comprehensive review of the current literature. *Pediatr Blood Cancer* 2009; 53(7):1171–9.

[10] Scarpa M, Bertin M, Ruffolo C, Polese L, D'Amico DF, Angriman I. A systematic review on the clinical diagnosis of gastrointestinal stromal tumors. *J Surg Oncol* 2008; 98(5):384–92.

[11] Kim KM, Kang DW, Moon WS, et al. Gastrointestinal stromal tumors in Koreans: it's incidence and the clinical, pathologic and immunohistochemical findings. *J Korean Med Sci* 2005; 20:977-84

[12] Pappo AS, Janeway KA. Pediatric gastrointestinal stromal tumors. *Hematol Oncol Clin North Am* 2009; 23(1):15–34–vii.

[13] Burgoyne AM, Somaiah N, Sicklick JK. Gastrointestinal stromal tumors in the setting of multiple tumor syndromes. *Curr Opin Oncol* 2014; 26(4):408–14.

[14] Postow MA, Robson ME. Inherited gastrointestinal stromal tumor syndromes: mutations, clinical features, and therapeutic implications. *Clin Sarcoma Res* 2012; 2(1):16.

[15] Lu-Emerson C, Plotkin SR. The Neurofibromatoses. Part 1: NF1. *Rev neurol Dis* 2009; 6(2):E47-53

[16] Miettinen M, Fetsch JF, Sobin LH, Lasota J. Gastrointestinal stromal tumors in patients with neurofibromatosis 1: a clinicopathologic and molecular genetic study of 45 cases. *Am J Surg Pathol.* 2006; 30(1):90–6.

[17] Carney JA, Stratakis CA. Familial paraganglioma and gastric stromal sarcoma: A new syndrome distinct from the Carney triad. *Am J Med Genet* 2002; 108(2):132–9.

[18] Stratakis CA, Carney JA. The triad of paragangliomas, gastric stromal tumours and pulmonary chondromas (Carney triad), and the dyad of paragangliomas and gastric stromal sarcomas (Carney-Stratakis syndrome): molecular genetics and clinical implications. *J Intern Med* 2009; 266(1):43–52.

[19] Pantaleo MA, Astolfi A, Indio V, et al. SDHA Loss-of-function mutations in KIT–PDGFRA wild-type gastrointestinal stromal tumors identified by massively parallel sequencing. *J Natl Cancer Inst* 2011; 103(12):983–7.

[20] Oyedotun KS, Lemire BD. The quaternary structure of the Saccharomyces cerevisiae succinate dehydrogenase. Homology modeling, cofactor docking, and molecular dynamics simulation studies. *J Biol Chem* 2004; 279(10):9424–31.
[21] Stiller CA. *Childhood cancer in Britain: incidence, survival, mortality.* Oxford University Press, Oxford, 2007.
[22] Janeway KA, Weldon CB. Pediatric gastrointestinal stromal tumor. *Semin Pediatr Surg* 2012; 21(1):31–43.
[23] Somerhausen N, Fletcher C. Gastrointestinal stromal tumours: an update. *Sarcoma* 1998; 2(3-4):133-41
[24] Mazur MT, Clark HB. Gastric stromal tumors. Reappraisal of histogenesis. *Am J Surg Pathol* 1983; 7(6):507–19.
[25] Hirota S, Isozaki K, Moriyama Y, et al. Gain-of-function mutations of c-kit in human gastrointestinal stromal tumors. *Science* 1998; 279(5350):577–80.
[26] Novelli M, Rossi S, Rodriguez-Justo M, et al. DOG1 and CD117 are the antibodies of choice in the diagnosis of gastrointestinal stromal tumours. *Histopathology* 2010; 57(2):259–70.
[27] Judson I. Gastrointestinal stromal tumours (GIST): biology and treatment. *Ann Oncol* 2002; 13(suppl 4):287–9.
[28] Fletcher CD, Berman JJ, Corless C, et al. Diagnosis of gastrointestinal stromal tumors: a consensus approach. *Int J Surg Pathol* 2002; 10(2):81–9.
[29] Miettinen M, Majidi M, Lasota J. Pathology and diagnostic criteria of gastrointestinal stromal tumors (GISTs): a review. *Eur J Cancer* 2002; 38 Suppl 5:S39–51.
[30] Reith JD, Goldblum JR, Lyles RH, Weiss SW. Extragastrointestinal (soft tissue) stromal tumors: an analysis of 48 cases with emphasis on histologic predictors of outcome. *Mod Pathol* 2000; 13(5):577–85.
[31] Singer S, Rubin BP, Lux ML, et al. Prognostic value of KIT mutation type, mitotic activity, and histologic subtype in gastrointestinal stromal tumors. *J Clin Oncol.* 2002; 20(18):3898–905.
[32] Corless CL, Barnett CM, Heinrich MC. Gastrointestinal stromal tumours: origin and molecular oncology. *Nat Rev Cancer* 2011; 11(12):865–78.
[33] Daniels M, Lurkin I, Pauli R, et al. Spectrum of KIT/PDGFRA/BRAF mutations and phosphatidylinositol-3-kinase pathway gene alterations in gastrointestinal stromal tumors (GIST). *Cancer Letters.* 2011; 312(1):43–54.

[34] Miettinen M, Lasota J. Gastrointestinal stromal tumors. *Gastroenterol Clin North Am* 2013; 42(2):399–415.
[35] Miettinen M, Makhlouf H, Sobin LH, Lasota J. Gastrointestinal stromal tumors of the jejunum and ileum: a clinicopathologic, immune-histochemical, and molecular genetic study of 906 cases before imatinib with long-term follow-up. *Am J Surg Pathol* 2006; 30(4):477–89.
[36] Miettinen M, Lasota J. Gastrointestinal stromal tumors: pathology and prognosis at different sites. *Semin Diagn Pathol* 2006; 23(2):70–83.
[37] DeMatteo RP, Lewis JJ, Leung D, Mudan SS, Woodruff JM, Brennan MF. Two hundred gastrointestinal stromal tumors: recurrence patterns and prognostic factors for survival. *Ann Surg* 2000; 231(1):51–8.
[38] Hohenberger P, Ronellenfitsch U, Oladeji O, et al. Pattern of recurrence in patients with ruptured primary gastrointestinal stromal tumour. *Br J Surg* 2010; 97(12):1854–9.
[39] Joensuu H, Rutkowski P, Nishida T, et al. KIT and PDGFRA mutations and the risk of GI stromal tumor recurrence. *J Clin Oncol* 2015; 33(6):634-42.
[40] Huang H-Y, Li C-F, Huang W-W, et al. A modification of NIH consensus criteria to better distinguish the highly lethal subset of primary localized gastrointestinal stromal tumors: A subdivision of the original high-risk group on the basis of outcome. *Surgery* 2007; 141(6):748–56.
[41] Gold JS, Gönen M, Gutiérrez A, et al. Development and validation of a prognostic nomogram for recurrence-free survival after complete surgical resection of localised primary gastrointestinal stromal tumour: a retrospective analysis. *Lancet Oncol* 2009; 10(11):1045–52.
[42] Joensuu H, Eriksson M, Sundby Hall K, et al. One vs three years of adjuvant imatinib for operable gastrointestinal stromal tumor: a randomized trial. *JAMA* 2012; 307(12):1265–72.
[43] Ando N, Goto H, Niwa Y, et al. The diagnosis of GI stromal tumors with EUS-guided fine needle aspiration with immunohistochemical analysis. *Gastrointest Endosc* 2002; 55(1):37–43.
[44] Chak A, Canto MI, Rösch T, et al. Endosonographic differentiation of benign and malignant stromal cell tumors. *Gastrointest Endosc* 1997; 45(6):468–73.
[45] National Comprehensive Cancer Network Clinical Practice Guidelines in Oncology: Soft Tissue Sarcoma. www.nccn.orgprofessional sphysicianglsPDFsarcoma.pdf. 2015. pp. 1–126.

[46] ESMO/European Sarcoma Network Working Group. Gastrointestinal stromal tumours: ESMO clinical practice guidelines for diagnosis, treatment and follow-up. *Ann Oncol* 2014; 25 suppl 3:iii21–26.

[47] Eriksson M, Reichardt P, Hall KS, et al. *Needle biopsy through the abdominal wall for the diagnosis of GIST – Does it pose any risk for tumor cell seeding and recurrence?* Abstract presentation, the Connective Tissue Oncology Meeting, Prague, 2012.

[48] DeMatteo RP, Maki RG, Singer S, Gönen M, Brennan MF, Antonescu CR. Results of tyrosine kinase inhibitor therapy followed by surgical resection for metastatic gastrointestinal stromal tumor. *Ann Surg*. 2007; 245(3):347–52.

[49] Raut CP, Posner M, Desai J, et al. Surgical management of advanced gastrointestinal stromal tumors after treatment with targeted systemic therapy using kinase inhibitors. *J Clin Oncol* 2006; 24(15):2325–31.

[50] Jones RL, McCall J, Adam A, et al. Radiofrequency ablation is a feasible therapeutic option in the multi-modality management of sarcoma. *Eur J Surg Oncol* 2010; 36(5):477–82.

[51] Plaat BE, Hollema H, Molenaar WM, et al. Soft tissue leiomyosarcomas and malignant gastrointestinal stromal tumors: differences in clinical outcome and expression of multidrug resistance proteins. *J Clin Oncol* 2000; 18(18):3211–20.

[52] Edmonson JH, Marks RS, Buckner JC, Mahoney MR. Contrast of response to dacarbazine, mitomycin, doxorubicin, and cisplatin (DMAP) plus GM-CSF between patients with advanced malignant gastrointestinal stromal tumors and patients with other advanced leiomyosarcomas. *Cancer Invest* 2002; 20(5-6):605–12.

[53] Demetri GD, Reichardt P, Kang YK, et al. Efficacy and safety of regorafenib for advanced gastrointestinal stromal tumours after failure of imatinib and sunitinib (GRID): an international, multicentre, randomised, placebo-controlled, phase 3 trial. *Lancet*. 2013; 381(9863):295–302.

[54] Demetri GD, van Oosterom AT, Garrett CR, et al. Efficacy and safety of sunitinib in patients with advanced gastrointestinal stromal tumour after failure of imatinib: a randomised controlled trial. *Lancet* 2006; 368(9544):1329–38.

In: Gastrointestinal Stromal Tumors in Adults … ISBN: 978-1-63483-679-1
Editor: Atif A. Ahmed

Chapter 2

MOLECULAR GENETICS

Gabriel Minarik*

Faculty of Medicine, Institute of Molecular Biomedicine,
Comenius University in Bratislava, Bratislava, Slovakia

ABSTRACT

Numerous advances were made in thelast decade in the research of gastrointestinal stromal tumors (GIST). The success in GIST diagnosis, therapy and prognosis was associated with discovery of mutations in the genes of two receptor tyrosine kinases, namely c-kit receptor tyrosine kinase (*KIT*) and platelet-derived growth factor receptor A (*PDGFRA*). Identified mutations were found to be the oncogenic drivers for GIST development and progression. A new and very promising therapeutic agent, imatinib mesylate, with a strong and specific inhibitory action on relevant receptor tyrosine kinases aberrant signaling, necessitated subsequent pilot therapies and clinical trials as a treatment for GIST. Unprecedented positive therapeutic responses were subsequently recorded and the successful targeted therapy story continued. It is now well known that mutations in the most relevant driver genes and recently identified genetic signatures play important roles in GIST diagnosis, staging, therapy, management and prognosis. Molecular analysis has become an inseparable part of the current personalized approach to clinical management of GIST patients.

* Email: gabriel.minarik@gmail.com

1. Introduction: Discovery of GIST Associated Genes

In the past, the diagnosis of GIST was difficult due to lack of specific diagnostic markers, and unclear cellular origin and molecular etiopathogenesis of tumor cells [1].

In 1998, Hirota et al. identified CD117 (KIT) expression as GIST-specific marker useful in immunohistochemistry (IHC) based diagnosis of GIST and revealed the presence of gain-of function mutations in a gene encoding KIT in most of the analyzed GIST tumors (5 of 6 samples) [2]. Moreover, in experiments with murine cells transfected with mutant *KIT* gene ligand, independent and constitutive activation of KIT was recorded. Few years before the inoculation of nude athymic mice with mutant KIT expressing cells had resulted in tumor development [3], the causality of *KIT* mutations for GIST development was considered as confirmed. Mutations in another receptor tyrosine kinase - the *PDGFRA*, were subsequently identified as mutually exclusive causative mutations in *KIT* mutation-negative GISTs [4]. According to recent original studies, activating mutations in *KIT* or *PDGFRA* are present in 85 - 90% of GISTs [5-7].

In the remaining 10 - 15% of cases (called as "wild-type GISTs"), the cause of tumor development is considered to be the result of different processes associated with known driver gene amplification or overexpression, mutations in different genes located downstream in the signaling cascade of KIT and PDGFRA (e.g., *RAS*, *BRAF*, *PIK3CA*), mutations in genes associated with succinate dehydrogenase (SDH) complex II function (e.g., *SDHA*), or mutations in genes specific for particular syndromes (e.g., *NF1*, *SDHB*). Although mutations in the above mentioned genes are considered as the most important driver mutations, other genetic events are necessary for tumor development and progression.

In 2000, Fukasawa et al. identified chromosomal losses on different chromosomes during tumor evolution with two being the most prevalent, -14q and -22q. In 2003, -1p was also added to the list [4, 8, 9]. These findings were confirmed in a more recent study in 2011 and the list was broadened with -19q and -15q [10].

2. NONSYNDROMIC GIST - GENES AND THEIR ONCOGENIC MUTATIONS

The vast majority of GISTs are nonsyndromic and are characterized by high frequency (up to 90%) of gain-of-function mutations in receptor tyrosine kinases, namely c-KIT (KIT) and platelet derived growth factor receptor α (PDGFRA). Only a small subset of nonsyndromic GIST cases is associated with mutations in other genes or their molecular cause is not known yet.

2.1. *KIT* and *PDGFRA* Genes, Protein Structure and Function

KIT and *PDGFRA* genes are located on the same chromosomal region of chromosome 4 (4q12) and their products show a high level of sequence and structural homology. The *KIT* gene (ENSG00000157404) occupies almost 83 kb of chromosome 4, encodes a transcript with 5.2 kb (ENST00000288135) and is composed of 21 exons, all of which are coding. The *PDGFRA* gene (ENSG00000134853) occupies 69 kb of chromosome 4, encodes a transcript with 6.5 kb (ENST00000257290) and is composed of 23 exons, 22 of which are coding as the first exon encodes 5´- untranslated region. The KIT and PDGFRA proteins contain 976 and 1089 amino acids respectively, and act in cell membrane as receptor tyrosine kinases (RTK) (www.ensembl.org, accessed on 2014/12/29).

KIT and PDGFRA belong to type III RTK family, that includes platelet derived growth factor receptor β (PDGFRB), macrophage colony-stimulating-factor receptor (CSFR1), and Fl cytokine receptor (FLT3) (Type III RTKs: PDGFR, CSFR, Kit, FLT3 receptor family, introduction. accessed on 2014/12/29. IUPHAR/BPS Guide to PHARMACOLOGY, http://www.guide topharmacology.org/GRAC/FamilyIntroductionForward?familyId=322).

Their corresponding natural ligands are stem cell factor (SCF) and platelet derived growth factor α (PDGFA), respectively. Their proteins are composed of 5 Ig-like extracellular domains, one transmembrane domain, one intracellular juxtamembrane regulatory domain and tyrosine kinase domain, which in KIT and PDGFRA is split to ATP binding and phosphotransferase subdomains. GIST-causal mutations of *KIT* and *PDGFRA* genes are clustered to particular exons (*KIT* exons 9, 11, 13 and 17 and *PDGFRA* exons 12, 14 and 18) which correspond to the extracellular, juxtamembrane and kinase domains of RTK (Figure 1) [11].

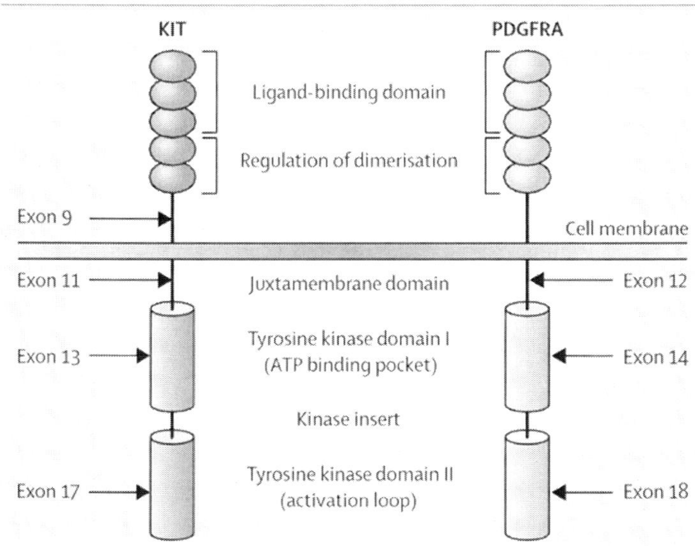

Figure 1. Structure of RTK III – KIT and PDGFRA, with information about localization of exons with known GIST-causal mutations [Reproduced with permission from Joensuu H, Hohenberger P, Corless CL. Gastrointestinal stromal tumour. Lancet 2013; 382(9896):973-83].

After binding of the ligand to the binding domain, structural changes abolish autoinhibitory function of the juxtamembrane domain, monomers of RTK homodimerize and autophosphorylation occurs at their tyrosine kinase domains.

The phosphorylation is then transferred further in intracellular signaling cascade when both KIT and PDGFRA use same downstream signaling pathways (Figure 2) containing RAS-RAF-MAPK, Src family kinases, PIK3CA-AKT and PLCγ [12]. In mutated KIT and PDGFRA, constitutive and ligand-independent autophosphorylation leads to activation of oncogenic transcription and deregulation of cell growth control.

2.2. Mutations in KIT and PDGFRA

2.2.1. Familial GIST- Heritable KIT and PDGFRA Mutations

Families with recurrent GISTs showing autosomal dominant trait of inheritance have been reported a decade before the association ofGIST and *KIT/PDGFRA* genes mutations was discovered [13]. Shortly thereafter, Hirota et al. and Heinrich et al. published results of identification of mutually exclusive mutations in *KIT* and *PDGFRA* genes identified in families with GIST history [2, 4]. Currently, there are known mutations in KIT exons 11, 13 and 17 (p.W557R, p.559_del, p.V559A; p.K642E; p.820Y) and PDGFRA exons 12 and 18 (p.V561D; p.D846Y). In patients with familial GIST other clinical features, like hyperpigmentation, urticaria pigmentosa, and dysphagia in *KIT* mutation-bearing patients or large hands, lipomas and small intestine fibrous tumors in *PDGFRA* mutation-bearing patients, were also identified [14-19]. The prevalence of germline *KIT* and *PDGFRA* genes mutations mimic their prevalence in sporadic GIST cases (see chapter 2.2.2.2). Syndromic GISTs were also identified as inherited diseases with germline mutations identified in genes *NF1* and *SDHB*, *SDHC* and *SDHD* or deletions of chromosomal locus containing *SDHB* gene (for more details about molecular genetics of syndromic GIST see chapter 2.3).

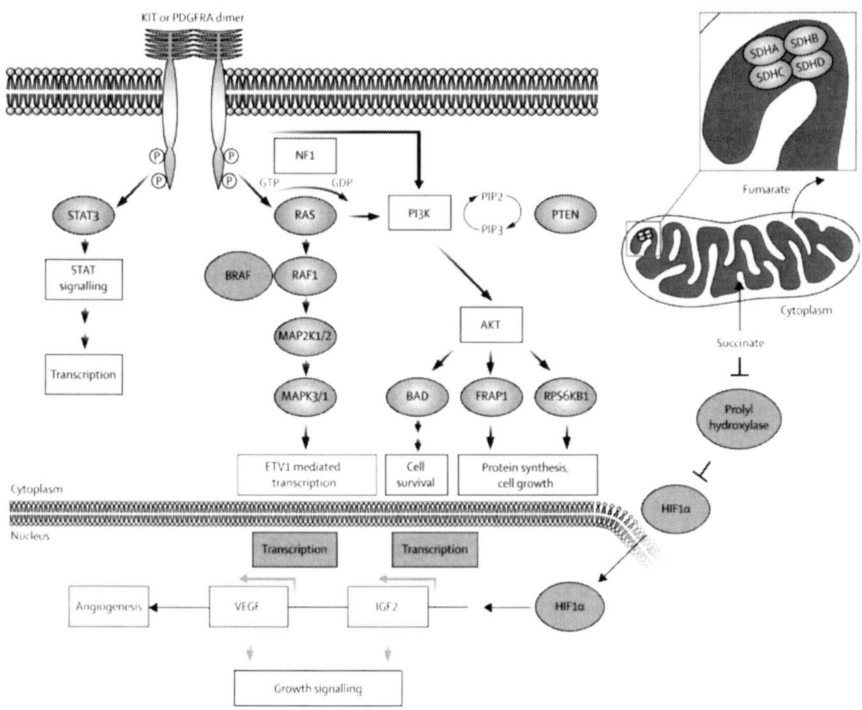

Figure 2. Downstream signaling pathway of activated KIT and PDGFRA [11].

2.2.2. Sporadic GIST– Primary KIT and PDGFRA Mutations

Mutations in KIT and PDGFRA receptor tyrosine kinases (RTK) are the most prevalent driver mutations in GIST patients with 85-90% prevalence on all sporadic GIST cases. In these, 70-85% are characterized by *KIT* and 5-15% by *PDGFRA* mutations [5-7, 20]. The mutations are not equally distributed in genes but are concentrated in specific exons. In GIST patients *KIT* mutations are concentrated in exon 9, 11, 13 and 17 and *PDGFRA* mutations in exons 12, 14 and 18. As the first exon of *PDGFRA* gene is non-coding, *KIT* exons 11, 13 and 17 are in fact corresponding to exons 12, 14 and 18 of *PDGFRA*. Surprisingly, frequencies of oncogenic mutations per exon in *KIT* and *PDGFRA* are not in concordance as *KIT* mutations occur most frequently in exon 11, less prevalently in exon 9 and only rarely identified in exons 13 and 17, while *PDGRA* is most frequently mutated in exon 18 and mutations in exons 12 and 14 are relatively rare.

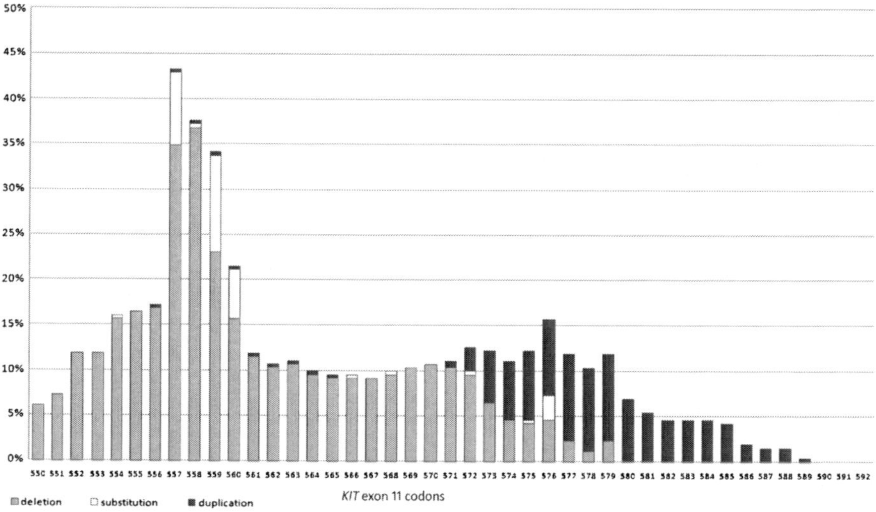

Figure 3. Frequency of KIT exon 11 codons affected by deletions, substitutions and/or tandem duplications [Reproduced with permission from: Wozniak A, Rutkowski P, Piskorz A, et al. Prognostic value of KIT/PDGFRA mutations in gastrointestinal stromal tumours (GIST): Polish Clinical GIST Registry Experience. Ann Oncol 2012; 23(2):353-60].

According to recently published data from population based studies frequencies of mutations per exons were between 60.9-63.2%, 5.5-8.3%, 1.2-1.4% and 0-0.6% in *KIT* exons 11, 9, 13 and 17, respectively. For *PDGFRA*, the frequencies varied between 7.6-12.0%, 2.0-3.4 and 0-1.1% in exon 18, 12 and 14 (out of 492 samples [5]; 87 patients [21]; and 278 samples [6]).

The most prevalent mutation types are in-frame deletions (approximately 40% of all *KIT* and *PDGFRA* mutations in GIST patients). Less prevalent are in-frame insertions and substitutions or combinations of these. In-frame deletions are typical mutations of *KIT* exon 11, with most frequently deleted amino acid positions 557-559 (Figure 3) [6, 7]. Of all in-frame deletions, the p.557_558del in *KIT* exon 11 has been identified as the most frequent. Nevertheless, because of the variable location and range of in-frame deletions in *KIT* exon 11, and if all mutations were counted together independently on their type, substitutions p.D842V in *PDGFRA* exon 18, p.V559D in KIT exon 11 and duplication (insertion) p. 502_503dup2 in KIT exon 9 would be considered as the most frequent single mutations [5, 6, 21] (Figure 4).

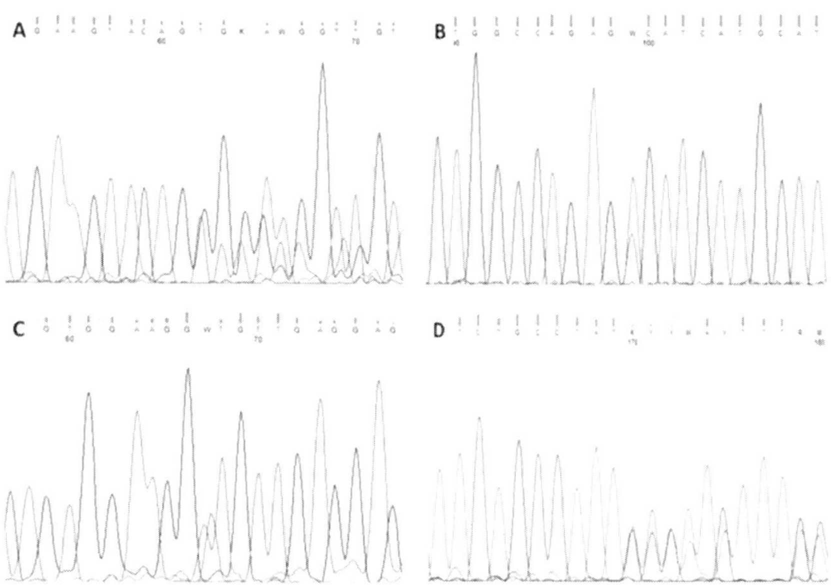

Figure 4. Most frequent mutations identified by Sanger sequencing in GIST patients: A) p.557_558del in KIT exon 11; B) p.D842V in PDGFRA exon 18; C) p.V559D in KIT exon 11 and D) p. 502_503dup2 in KIT exon 9.

When Emile et al. compared frequencies of the ten most frequent mutations identified in their population-based study with known data from SWOGS0033 and EORTC92006 studies that were based on analysis of GIST patients with advanced GIST, significant differences were identified in 6 of them [5]. Identified differences in mutation frequencies were in concordance with the different impact of particular mutations on GIST progression and prognosis. In patients with advanced GIST, the most prevalent mutations were more frequent in those with worse prognosis (e.g., p. 557_558del in *KIT* exon 11, p. 502_503dup2 in *KIT* exon 9).

2.3. *PIK3CA*, *RAS*, *BRAF* and *SDHA* Mutations

It was hypothesized that in patients with and without *KIT* and *PDGFRA* oncogenic mutations causal mutations in signaling molecules located downstream in RTK signaling cascade could be oncogenic drivers. These could be considered not only as oncogenic drivers but also as potential modifiers of disease progression and targeted therapy utility. The known oncogenes, PIK3CA, RAS and BRAF, play important roles in the KIT signaling cascade (Figure 2). In all three genes, mutational hot-spots were identified in previous studies (V600E of BRAF; E542K, E545K, or H1047R in *PIK3CA*; and codons 12 and 13 mutations in *KRAS*) and their oncogenic effect was confirmed [22-24].

2.3.1. BRAF Gene Mutations

The BRAF oncogenic mutation, V600E, is known as the most prevalent oncogenic mutation in melanoma [22]. In a small subset of melanoma cases, *KIT* mutations were also found as mutually exclusive [25]. Thus it is hypothesized that BRAF mutations could also be oncogenic in GIST patients without *KIT* and *PDGFRA* mutations. In recently published studies, V600E mutation was found in 3.5-13% of adult GIST patients lacking *KIT* and *PDGFRA* mutations [21, 26-28]. Moreover, it was detected as secondary mutation in patients with acquired imatinib resistance. Therefore it is considered, although rare, that it could represent an alternative mechanism of secondary imatinib resistance in GIST [26].

2.3.2. PIK3CA Gene Mutations

A mutation in *PIK3CA*, H1047L, was later found in a small percentage of tumor cells of patient bearing in-frame deletion in *KIT* exon 11 [21]. The H1047 amino acid position is highly conserved and the H1047L mutation is functionally similar to another frequently identified hot-spot oncogenic mutation in cancer patients, i.e., H1047R [23]. Moreover, the H1047L *PIK3CA* mutation is found to be present in low frequency in breast cancer patients [29]. Recently, in one GIST patient without *KIT* or *PDGFRA* mutations, a *BRAF* gene V600E primary mutation was identified. After targeted therapy with BRAF inhibitor and short term therapy success, the disease progressed and secondary *PIK3CA* oncogenic mutation H1047R was identified in one of three metastatic lesions tested. Therefore, secondary mutation screening in *PIK3CA* could also be considered in cases where the primary or secondary chosen targeted therapy fails to inhibit tumor progression [30].

2.3.3. KRAS Gene Mutations

In 2012, the original study of Miranda et al. was the first to report *KRAS* mutations in GIST patients with *KIT* and *PDGFRA* mutations. They detected that 5% and 2% of naïve GIST patients carry concomitant *KRAS* and *BRAF* mutations. In subsequent in vitro functional studies on cells bearing imatinib sensitive *KIT* mutation and concomitant *KRAS* and *BRAF* oncogenic mutations, primary resistance to imatinib treatment was recorded. Therefore it was hypothesized that presence of such *KRAS* and *BRAF* mutations could be responsible for unexpected primary resistance in samples with *KIT* and *PDGFRA* imatinib sensitive mutations which were identified in previously performed clinical studies [31]. However these results were not confirmed in a large cohort study performed on 514 GIST samples where no *KRAS* mutations were found [32]. According to most recent results the frequency of *KRAS* mutations should be below 0.3% thus not playing an important role in disease progression or primary and secondary resistance to imatinib treatment in patients with imatinib sensitive *KIT* and *PDGFRA* mutations [32, 33].

2.3.4. SDHA Gene Mutations

Most recently, novel loss-of-function mutations in the *SDHA* gene were found by whole exome sequencing of pediatric and young adult GIST patients without *KIT* and *PDGFRA* mutations. The germline mutation p.R31X was found in one of six patients and p.D38V mutation was identified in larger panel of 11 pediatric and young adult patients. Genetic mutations and loss of immunohistochemical expression of *SDHA* and *SDHB* were both detected in tumor tissue of *SDHA* mutation-bearing samples, while in the remaining tumors without *SDHA* mutations only immunohistochemical loss of *SDHB* expression was present [34]. The possibility to use *SDHA*-based immunohistochemistry to identify *SDHA* mutation-bearing GISTs was later confirmed in subsequent studies, where also other novel *SDHA* gene mutations (e.g., p.Q54X, p.T267M, c.1663 + 3G > C) were identified [35, 36].

2.4. Genotype – Phenotype Correlations of KIT and PDGFRA Mutations in GIST Patients

2.4.1. Pre-Imatinib Era

With the identification of GIST oncogenic mutations in *KIT* and *PDGFRA*, it was hypothesized that different oncogenic mutations may lead to different tumor phenotypes.

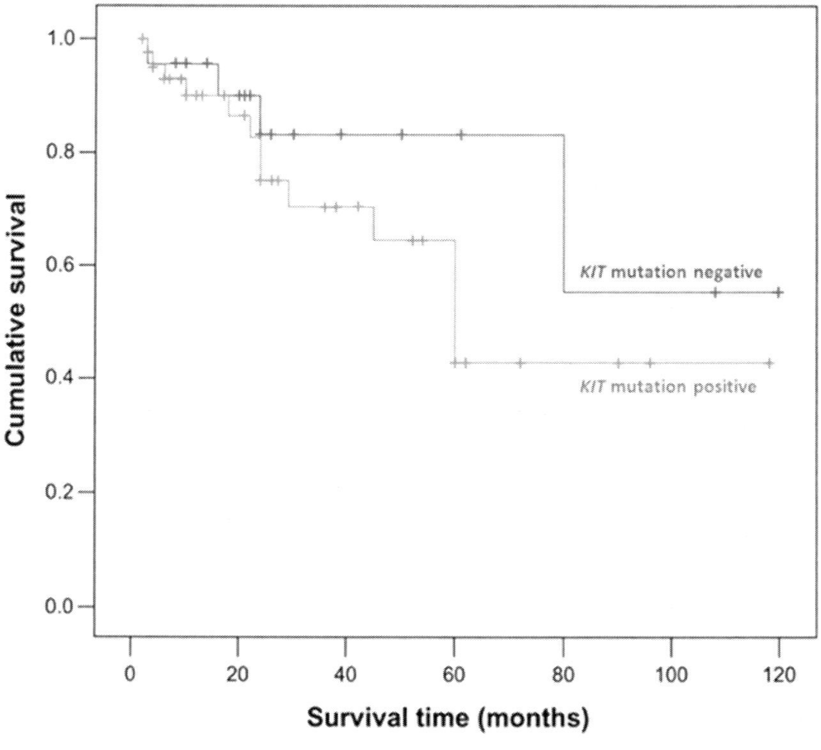

Figure 5. Kaplan–Meier survival-curve analysis in patients with positive and negative c-KIT mutation [Reproduced with permission from: Ma YY, Yu S, He XJ, et al. Involvement of c-KIT mutation in the development of gastrointestinal stromal tumors through proliferation promotion and apoptosis inhibition. Onco Targets Ther 2014; 7:637-43].

In the study of Ernst et al, based on the analysis of *KIT* exon 11 mutational status of 35 patients with gastric GISTs, the association between *KIT* exon 11 mutations and decreased survival was detected ($p = 0.001$), when 30% of patients with mutation, vs. 65% patients without mutation, survived more than

3 years, respectively [37]. These findings were confirmed in a later study with similar design based on analysis of 124 GIST patients. In *KIT* exon 11 mutation-bearing patients the tumor size was larger, tumor cells showed higher mitotic counts and more necrosis, and hemorrhage was found within the tumors. Moreover, mutation-positive GISTs showed more frequent recurrences ($p = 0.0005$) and had higher mortality ($p = 0.0001$) than the mutation-negative GISTs [38] (Figure 5).

2.4.2. Post Imatinib Era

After first succesfull therapies of metastatic GIST patients with imatinib mesylate it was hypothesized that differencies in clinical response on imatinib treatment could be caused by differencies in oncogenic mutations (different types of mutations in different exons of different genes) [40]. In 2003, a clinical study combined with *in vitro* experiments confirmed genotype-phenotype correlations between *KIT* and *PDGFRA* mutational status and predicted disease prognosis or therapy response (Figure 6) [20]. In this study performed on 127 tumor specimens, patients with exon 11 mutant KIT protein benefit at most from treatment with imatinib mesylate. They reached partial response (PR) in 83.5%, while patients whose tumors expressed either an exon 9 mutant isoform protein or contained no detectable mutation of *KIT* or *PDGFRA* had significantly lower PR rates of 47.8% ($p = 0.0006$) and 0.0% ($p < 0.0001$), respectively. The frequency of PR was also significantly different between patients with an exon 9 mutation versus patients with no detectable *KIT* and *PDGFRA* mutation ($p = 0.013$). However, there was no statistically significant difference in the response rates between the group of patients with *KIT* exon 11 point mutations and the group with exon 11 deletion mutations or between the group with heterozygous tumors and the group with tumors homozygous/hemizygous for exon 11 deletion mutations. After logistical regression analysis, the presence of a *KIT* exon 11 mutation was identified as the strongest predictor of response (hazard ratio (HR), 7.85; 95% CI, 3.55 to 17.37). In the same study, *in vitro* experiments revealed that the Chinese hamster ovary cells expressing *KIT* with most frequent *KIT* mutations in exons 11, 9, 13 and 17 showed sensitivity to "standard" dose of imatinib, while most frequent *PDGFRA* mutation D842V expressing cells needed 10- to 20-times higher concentration for similar rate of phosporylation inhibition. These finding were in agreement with presence of two patients, bearing *PDGFRA* D842V mutations, who were resistant (primary resistance) to imatinib treatment in the clinical arm of the study while patients with different *PDGFRA* mutations showed similar response rated as patients with *KIT* mutations [20]. Later on, the association between presence of deletion of Trp-557 and Lys-558 (p.557_558del in *KIT* exon 11) in the juxtamembrane domain of the KIT and metastatic behavior of tumor was identified in the study of 55 sporadic GIST patiens [41].

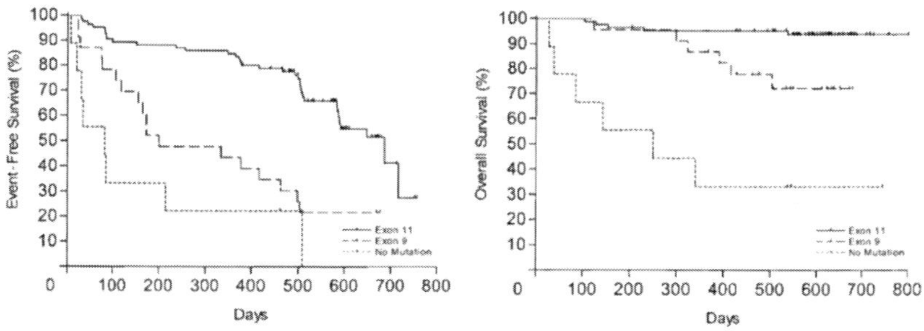

Figure 6. Gastrointestinal stromal tumor kinase genotype correlation with event-free and overall survival in patients bearing KIT exon 11, KIT exon 9 and without mutations in the two mentioned exons treated with "standard" dose (400 mg per day) of imatinib [Reproduced with permission from: Heinrich MC, Corless CL, Demetri GD, et al. Kinase mutations and imatinib response in patients with metastatic gastrointestinal stromal tumor. J Clin Oncol 2003; 21(23):4342-9].

In 2006 and 2008, other phase III clinical trials managed by EORTC and SWOG were also evaluated. Thanks to larger patient groups, analysis on 377 and 428 patients, with focus on potential correlation between *KIT* and *PDGFRA* mutation status and disease progression or therapy success, confirmed previous findings and identified novel associations. In the study from 2006, the poor response to therapy with standard dose of imatinib in *KIT* exon 9 mutation-bearing patients was detected. *KIT* exon 9 mutation was found to be the strongest adverse prognostic factor for response to imatinib. It increased the relative risk of progression by 171% ($p < 0.0001$) and the relative risk of death by 190% ($p < 0.0001$) when compared with *KIT* exon 11 mutations. Similarly, the relative risk of progression was increased by 108% ($p < 0.0001$) and the relative risk of death by 76% ($p = 0.028$) in patients without detectable *KIT* or *PDGFRA* mutations. Moreover, when two dosage regimes were compared – 400 mg (standard dose) and 800 mg (high dose) of imatinib per day, the *KIT* exon 9 mutation-bearing patients showed significantly superior progression-free survival ($p = 0.0013$), with a reduction of the relative risk of about 61% when treated with high dose of imatinib [42].

Later in the 2008 study, analysis of 428 patients, with similar design - genotype-phenotype correlation and dosage regimes of 400 and 800 mg of imatinib per day comparison, was performed with almost concordant results. The presence of *KIT* exon 11 mutation genotype correlated with improved treatment outcome when compared with *KIT* exon 9 mutation and wild-type genotypes on standard dose treatment. Complete response/partial response ratio (CR/PR) was 71.7% vs. 44.4% (p = 0.007) vs. 44.6% (p = 0.0002), respectively. When time to tumor progression was compared, medians of 24.7 vs. 16.7 vs. 12.8 months and overall survival medians of 60.0 vs. 38.4 vs. 49.0 months were recorded, respectively. In contrast, survival outcomes for patients with *KIT* exon 9 mutations, *KIT* exon 11 mutations or WT GISTs were not affected by imatinib dose, but there was evidence of improved response rates for patients with *KIT* exon 9 mutation treated with imatinib 800 mg versus 400 mg - CR/PR = 67% *v* 17% (p = 0.02) [43]. This was confirmed in a recently published results of meta-analysis based on combined data of the previously mentioned trials from 2006 and 2008. The worse prognosis was confirmed for patients with wild type GIST, *KIT* exon 9 mutation or patients with other mutations if compared to *KIT* exon 11 mutation. Also the high dose treatment with imatinib resulted in significantly longer progression-free survival (PFS) for patients with *KIT* exon 9 mutations – estimated HR = 0.89 (p = 0.04), but without significant difference of overall survival (OS) and best overall response (Figure 7) [44].

In two of recent studies, the most frequent particular mutations or mutation types and their association with malignant potential or disease progression were compared. When 9 most frequent GIST mutations and deletions of *PDGFRA* exon 18 (PDGFRAex18del) and their prognostic value were compared, patients with *KIT* exon 9 p.502-503dup, *KIT* exon 11 p.557-558del, *KIT* exon 11 p.V559G and PDGFRAex18del were at high risk of malignancy. Mutations *PDGFRA* exon 18 p.D842V, *KIT* exon 11 p.W557R, *KIT* exon 11 p.V559D and *KIT* exon 11 p.L576P were of low risk and mutations *KIT* exon 11 p.V560D and *KIT* exon 11 p.560del were of very low risk malignancy [7, 45]. The longer relapse-free survival (RFS) was associated with substitutions in comparison to deletions and, from all genotypes, the shortest RFS was recorded in patients with p. 557_558del in *KIT* exon 11 (p = 0.001) [7]. Thus the malignant potential of the tumor could be the result of distinctive expression profiles influenced partially by presence of different *KIT* and *PDGFRA* mutations and partially by localization of tumor. In gene expression profiling studies, the clustering, according to the mutation type and according to tumor localization, was apparent [46, 47].

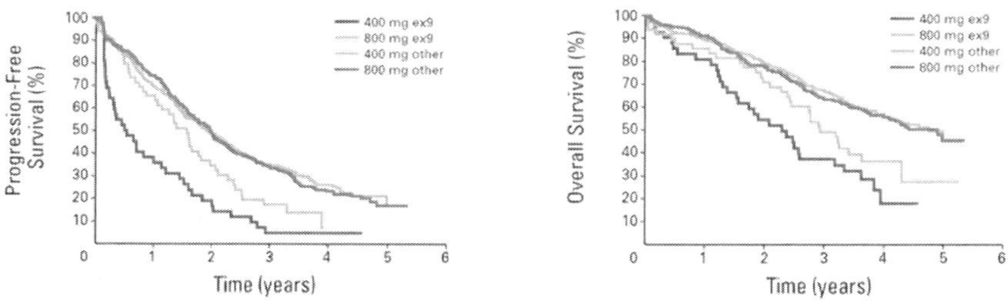

Figure 7. Progression-free survival and overall survival of GIST patients treated with standard and high dose of imatinig with focus on presence of KIT exon 9 (ex9) mutations; O – events, N – number of patients [Reproduced with permission from: Gastrointestinal Stromal Tumor Meta-Analysis Group (MetaGIST). Comparison of two doses of imatinib for the treatment of unresectable or metastatic gastrointestinal stromal tumors: a meta-analysis of 1,640 patients. J Clin Oncol 2010; 28(7):1247-53].

2.4.3. Secondary Mutations in KIT and PGFRA and Imatinib Treatment Efficacy

Soon after beginning of first clinical studies with imatinib treatment of GIST, the correlation between *KIT* and *PDGFRA* mutational status and response to imatinib treatment was identified. Together, subsets of patients showing primary resistance based on previously mentioned molecular characteristics of tumors (see chapter 2.4.2.2) and secondary (acquired) resistance to imatinib treatment were detected. In 2004, the first report of secondary resistance causing mutations found in *KIT* exon 13 was published. Surprisingly, all 5 patients in whom secondary resistance developed after imatinib treatment had the same mutation, *KIT* exon 13 p.V654A, that was not published in association with GIST before and was not previously present in the primary tumors of these patients. The other arguments for its resistance causality were that, it was present on the originally mutated imatinib sensitive allele (*cis*-position) and that its position in the KIT protein was in close proximity to imatinib contact points [48]. Later on, in vitro analysis of selected secondary mutations found in GIST patients confirmed its imatinib resistance nature [49]. In other studies, secondary resistance-causing mutations were also found in *KIT* exon 14 (e.g., p.T670I), *KIT* exon 17 (e.g., p.D820Y, p.N822K), *PDGFRA* exon 14 (e.g., p.H687Y) and *PDGFRA* exon 18 (e.g., p.D842V) [49-54]. In concordance with clonal evolution of cancer metastasis, multiple secondary mutations were reported in different metastatis, with unique secondary mutations per metastasis in single patients [52, 54].

2.4.4. *Sunitinib Efficacy in GIST Patients with KIT and PDGFRA Mutations*

For patients with unresectable GISTs resistant to treatment with imatinib, alternative RTK inhibitor was needed. The clinical trial from 2006, which evaluated GIST therapy with a novel multi-targeted receptor tyrosine kinase inhibitor, revealed that sunitinib malate was able to prolong time to tumor progression 4 times in comparison with placebo (27.3 vs. 6.4 weeks, $p < 0.0001$). Even more important findings were that in subset of imatinib resistant or intolerant patients, sunitinib reached similar objective response rate as in imatinib naïve GIST patients [55].

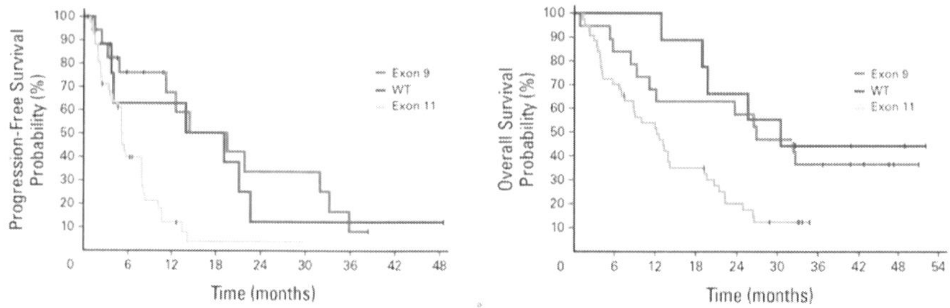

Figure 8. Impact of primary KIT genotype (KIT exon 9 mutations, KIT exon 11 mutations and no KIT exon 9 or 11 mutations - WT) on efficacy of sunitinib treatment presented as A) progression-free and B) overall survival [Reproduced with permission from: Heinrich MC, Maki RG, Corless CL, et al. Primary and secondary kinase genotypes correlate with the biological and clinical activity of sunitinib in imatinib-resistant gastrointestinal stromal tumor. J Clin Oncol 2008; 26(33): 5352-9].

Based on these results sunitinib was approved as effective treatment alternative for patients intolerant or resistant to imatinib therapy. In a subsequent clinical trial with imatinib resistant GIST and identified *KIT* and *PDGFRA* mutational status, correlation between tumor genotype and sunitinib therapy outcome was revealed. The highest clinical benefit rate (CBR) of 58% was recorded in patients with *KIT* exon 9 mutations, a similar CBR of 56% was recorded in patients with wild type *KIT* and *PDGFRA,* and the lowest CBR of 34% was recorded in patients with *KIT* exon 11 mutations. Patients with *PDGFRA* mutation showed no clinical benefit from sunitinib treatment. Similar results were gained when objective response rates (37% vs. 5%, $p = 0.002$), progression-free survival (19.4 months vs. 5.1 months, $p = 0.0005$) and median overall survival (OS) (26.9 months vs. 12.3 months) were compared between *KIT* exon 9 and *KIT* exon 11 mutation subsets. The *KIT* and *PDGFRA* wildtype patients showed similar results as patients with *KIT* exon 9 (Figure 8) [49].

2.4.5. Secondary Mutations in KIT and PGFRA and Imatinib Treatment Efficacy

In the study of Heinrich et al, sunitib second-line therapy outcome was evaluated in subset of patients bearing secondary mutations. In patients with secondary mutations in *KIT* exons 13 and 14, median PFS was significantly longer if compared to patients with *KIT* exons 17 and 18 secondary mutations (7.8 months vs. 2.3 months, p = 0.0157). Similarly, median OS was longer in *KIT* exon 13 and 14 mutations subset than for *KIT* exon 17 and 18 mutations subset but the difference was not statistically significant (13.0 months vs. 4.0 months, p = 0.160). In *in vitro* experiments of sunitinib effectivity of kinase phosphorylation inhibition, *KIT* and PDGFRA secondary mutations *KIT* exon 13 p.V654A and *KIT* exon 14 p.T670I were sunitinib sensitive and imatinib resistant. Analyzed secondary mutations in *KIT* exon 17 and 18 (p.D816H, p.D820G, p.N822K, p. Y823D and p.A829P) and *PDGFRA* exon 18 (p.D842V) were sunitinib as well as imatinib resistant [49].

2.4.6. Association between Mutations in KIT and PDGFRA and Tumor Localization

As revealed by independent studies, specific *KIT* and *PDGFRA* mutations were found to be associated with specific localization of GIST. The mutation *KIT* exon 9 p. 502_503dup2 was found to be associated with intestinal localization, while PDGFRA exon 18 p.D842V mutation was associated with gastric localization. These findings are in agreement with general clinic-pathological features of intestinal and gastric GIST and the malignant potential of these two mutations, as intestinal GISTs and GISTs with *KIT* exon 9 p. 502_503dup2 mutation have higher malignant potential as well as worse prognosis when compared with gastric GISTs and GISTs with *PDGFRA* exon 18 p.D842V mutation [5-7, 56].

2.5. Other Genetic Changes Associated with GIST Progression

Mutations of the previously mentioned genes in KIT/PDGFRA signaling cascade, although most important, are not the only genetic changes responsible for GIST development and transition from benign to malignant disease. According to the results of first original studies based on karyotyping and fluorescence in situ hybridization analyses, half to two-thirds of GISTs demonstrated monosomy/partial loss of chromosomes 14/14q and 22/22q, and these were identified in KIT as well as PDGFRA mutated GISTs [4, 8, 9, 57]. Later, although less frequent overall but more exclusive for malignant GIST, changes represented by loss of 1p, 9p, 11p and gain of 17p and 8q were identified [4, 10, 58, 59].

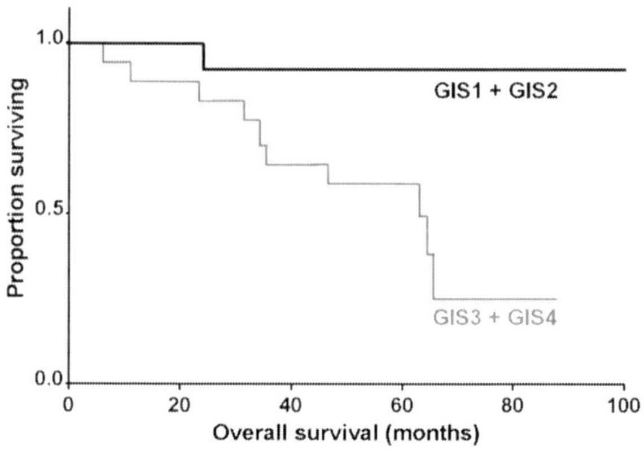

Figure 9. Different overall survival of patients classified according to alternative GIS staging system, GIS1 and 2 represents early-stage GISTs with good prognosis and GIS3 and 4 late-stage GISTs with worse prognosis [10].

In studies on candidate genes identification, other genes, located in loci considered as important for GIST development and benign to malignant progression, were identified. Deletions on 14q included the candidate genes *PARP2*, *APEX1* and *NDRG2* and *SIVA*, and in the deleted region on 22q, the *NF2* gene was localized. The gene *CDKN2A/2B* was identified at 9p, *ENO1* at 1p, and *MYC* at 8q [59]. In recent study, based on comparative analysis of primary GIST and primary leiomyosarcoma tumors, a different classification of GIST, independent on alternative to classical clinical staging, based on genetic changes was presented and named as Genomic Instability Stage - GIS. Authors were able to identify 4 stages of GIST that correlated well with disease progression, as GIS1 and 2 represented early-stage GISTs with good prognosis, while GIS3 and 4 late-stage GISTs with significantly worse prognosis ($p = 0.006$) (Figure 9) [10].

The 4 stages (from 1 to 4) were defined by increasing rate of *KIT* mutations, decrease of patient survival and accumulation of specific chromosomal aberrations. These aberrations were loss of distal part of chromosomes 1p, 19, 22q; loss of 14q; loss of proximal part of 1p, 15q and loss of chromosome 10 for GIS 1, 2, 3 and 4. When the impact of these chromosomal changes on specific cellular pathways was evaluated at shift between stages, GIS1 to GIS2-impaired apoptotic, DNA repair, and damage-response pathways, GIS2 to GIS3-affected mitotic cell cycle, and growth pathways and GIS3 to GIS4-impaired cell-cell adhesion and chromosomal organization pathways were identified [10].

3. Syndromic GIST - Genes and Their Oncogenic Mutations

There are three known syndromes with recurrent development of GIST as part of the disease – neurofibromatosis type 1 (NF1), Carney triad (CT) and Carney-Stratakis syndrome (CSS). All are responsible for small proportion of GIST and they are characterized by specific molecular alteration, which are not yet well defined in comparison to nonsyndromic GIST.

3.1. Neurofibromatosis Type 1

In less than 10% of patients with type 1 neurofibromatosis (NF1), who typically bear mutations in *NF1* gene, one or multiple GISTs will develop. According to the microscopic evaluation, these GISTs are of low-risk category with predominant intestinal localization. NF1 associated GISTs are characterized by CD117 (KIT) positivity by immunohistochemistry although originally no mutations in *KIT* and *PDGFRA* were detected in patients with NF1. Thus, different pathogenic mechanism for GIST development was considered [60, 61]. Nevertheless, in later studies, a small proportion of NF1 patients carried GISTs with *KIT* mutations [62, 63]. Furthermore, chromosomal aberrations which were frequently found in nonsyndromic GISTs less than 1 cm in size were detected frequently in GISTs of NF1 patients. These were represented by losses of 14q and 22q and were present in 87.5% and 41.7% of tumors in a small scale study [64]. Currently there is no detailed information about the molecular processes leading to development of GIST in NF1 patients.

3.2. Carney Triad and Carney-Stratakis Syndrome

In small subset of GISTs, which developed in young age patients with female predilection and predominant gastric localization, loss of expression of succinate dehydrogenase subunit B (SDHB) was recently detected as specific marker for immunohistochemistry [65]. These patients suffer from Carney triad (CT) or Carney-Stratakis syndrome (CSS) and together with multifocal GISTs, paraganglioma and pulmonary chondroma or paraganglioma will also develop, respectively. In both syndromes no *KIT* and *PDGFRA* mutations were detected in tumor samples. In mutational screening, no *SDHB*, *SDHC* and *SDHD* mutations were identified in CT patients. However, comparative genomic hybridization in CT patients revealed the recurrent chromosomal 1q12-q21 deletion, where the *SDHB* gene is localized [66]. On the other hand, in patients with CSS, characterized by autosomal dominant inheritance of disease, occurrence of loss-of-function germline mutations in *SDHB*, *SDHC* and *SDHD* was detected in the majority of patients in the original study (8 of 11 patients) [67]. The similarity between GISTs of CT and CSS patients, is not only in common genetic changes, but also in other clinical parameters, as they share epitheloid morphology predominance, frequent lymph node metastases, serial tumor occurence and unpredictable behavior [68].

REFERENCES

[1] Miettinen M, Lasota J. Histopathology of gastrointestinal stromal tumor. *J. Surg. Oncol.* 2011; 104(8): 865-873.

[2] Hirota S, Isozaki K, Moriyama Y, et al. Gain-of-function mutations of c-kit in human gastrointestinal stromal tumors. *Science* 1998; 279(5350): 577-580.

[3] Hashimoto K, Tsujimura T, Moriyama Y, et al. Transforming and differentiation-inducing potential of constitutively activated c-kit mutant genes in the IC-2 murine interleukin-3-dependent mast cell line. *Am. J. Pathol.* 1996; 148(1):189-200.

[4] Heinrich MC, Corless CL, Duensing A, et al. PDGFRA activating mutations in gastrointestinal stromal tumors. *Science,* 2003. 299(5607):708-710.

[5] Emile JF, Brahimi S, Coindre JM, et al. Frequencies of KIT and PDGFRA mutations in the MolecGIST prospective population-based

study differ from those of advanced GISTs. *Med. Oncol.* 2012; 29(3):1765-72.

[6] Minarik G, Plank L, Lasabová Z, et al. Spectrum of mutations in gastrointestinal stromal tumor patients - a population-based study from Slovakia. *APMIS;* 2013. 121(6):539-48.

[7] Wozniak A, Rutkowski P, Piskorz A, et al. Prognostic value of KIT/PDGFRA mutations in gastrointestinal stromal tumours (GIST): Polish Clinical GIST Registry experience. *Ann. Oncol.* 2012; 23(2):353-60.

[8] Fukasawa T, Chong JM, Sakurai S, et al. Allelic loss of 14q and 22q, NF2 mutation, and genetic instability occur independently of c-kit mutation in gastrointestinal stromal tumor. *Jpn J. Cancer Res.* 2000; 91(12): 1241-9.

[9] Gunawan B, Bergmann F, Höer J, et al. Biological and clinical significance of cytogenetic abnormalities in low-risk and high-risk gastrointestinal stromal tumors. *Hum. Pathol.* 2002; 33(3):316-21.

[10] Ylipaa A, Hunt KK, Yang J, et al. Integrative genomic characterization and a genomic staging system for gastrointestinal stromal tumors. *Cancer* 2011; 117(2):380-9.

[11] Joensuu H, Hohenberger P, Corless CL. Gastrointestinal stromal tumour. *Lancet* 2013; 382(9896):973-83.

[12] Roskoski R Jr. Structure and regulation of Kit protein-tyrosine kinase--the stem cell factor receptor. *Biochem. Biophys. Res. Commun.* 2005; 338(3):1307-15.

[13] Marshall JB, Diaz-Arias AA, Bochna GS, Vogele KA. Achalasia due to diffuse esophageal leiomyomatosis and inherited as an autosomal dominant disorder. Report of a family study. *Gastroenterology* 1990; 98(5 Pt 1):1358-65.

[14] Nishida T, Hirota S, Taniguchi M, et al. Familial gastrointestinal stromal tumours with germline mutation of the KIT gene. *Nat. Genet.* 1998; 19(4):323-4.

[15] Beghini A, Tibiletti MG, Roversi G, et al., Germline mutation in the juxtamembrane domain of the kit gene in a family with gastrointestinal stromal tumors and urticaria pigmentosa. *Cancer* 2001; 92(3):657-62.

[16] Maeyama H, Hidaka E, Ota H, et al. Familial gastrointestinal stromal tumor with hyperpigmentation: association with a germline mutation of the c-kit gene. *Gastroenterology* 2001; 120(1):210-5.

[17] Isozaki K, Terris B, Belghiti J, et al. Germline-activating mutation in the kinase domain of KIT gene in familial gastrointestinal stromal tumors. *Am. J. Pathol.* 2000; 157(5):1581-5.

[18] Pasini B, Matyakhina L, Bei T, et al. Multiple gastrointestinal stromal and other tumors caused by platelet-derived growth factor receptor alpha gene mutations: a case associated with a germline V561D defect. *J. Clin. Endocrinol. Metab.* 2007; 92(9):3728-32.

[19] Chompret A, Kannengiesser C, Barrois M, et al. PDGFRA germline mutation in a family with multiple cases of gastrointestinal stromal tumor. *Gastroenterology* 2004; 126(1):318-21.

[20] Heinrich MC, Corless CL, Demetri GD, et al. Kinase mutations and imatinib response in patients with metastatic gastrointestinal stromal tumor. *J. Clin. Oncol.* 2003; 21(23):4342-9.

[21] Daniels M, Lurkin I, Pauli R, et al. Spectrum of KIT/PDGFRA/BRAF mutations and Phosphatidylinositol-3-Kinase pathway gene alterations in gastrointestinal stromal tumors (GIST). *Cancer Lett.* 2011; 312(1):43-54.

[22] Davies H, Bignell GR, Cox C, et al. Mutations of the BRAF gene in human cancer. *Nature* 2002; 417(6892):949-54.

[23] Kang S, Bader AG, Vogt PK. Phosphatidylinositol 3-kinase mutations identified in human cancer are oncogenic. *Proc. Natl. Acad. Sci. USA* 2005; 102(3):802-7.

[24] Wan PT, Garnett MJ, Roe SM, et al. Mechanism of activation of the RAF-ERK signaling pathway by oncogenic mutations of B-RAF. *Cell* 2004; 116(6):855-67.

[25] Willmore-Payne C, Holden JA, Tripp S, Layfield LJ. Human malignant melanoma: detection of BRAF- and c-kit-activating mutations by high-resolution amplicon melting analysis. *Hum. Pathol.*, 2005. 36(5): p. 486-93.

[26] Agaram NP, Wong GC, Guo T, et al. Novel V600E BRAF mutations in imatinib-naive and imatinib-resistant gastrointestinal stromal tumors. *Genes Chromosomes Cancer* 2008; 47(10):853-9.

[27] Agaimy A, Terracciano LM, Dirnhofer S, et al. V600E BRAF mutations are alternative early molecular events in a subset of KIT/PDGFRA wild-type gastrointestinal stromal tumours. *J. Clin. Pathol.* 2009; 62(7):613-6.

[28] Hostein I, Faur N, Primois C, et al. BRAF mutation status in gastrointestinal stromal tumors. *Am. J. Clin. Pathol.* 2010; 133(1):141-8.

[29] Stemke-Hale K, Gonzalez-Angulo AM, Lluch A, et al. An integrative genomic and proteomic analysis of PIK3CA, PTEN, and AKT mutations in breast cancer. *Cancer Res.* 2008; 68(15):6084-91.

[30] Falchook GS, Trent JC, Heinrich MC, et al. BRAF mutant gastrointestinal stromal tumor: first report of regression with BRAF inhibitor dabrafenib (GSK2118436) and whole exomic sequencing for analysis of acquired resistance. *Oncotarget* 2013; 4(2):310-5.

[31] Miranda C, Nucifora M, Molinari F, et al. KRAS and BRAF mutations predict primary resistance to imatinib in gastrointestinal stromal tumors. *Clin. Cancer Res.* 2012; 18(6):1769-76.

[32] Lasota J, Xi L, Coates T, et al. No KRAS mutations found in gastrointestinal stromal tumors (GISTs): molecular genetic study of 514 cases. *Mod. Pathol.* 2013; 26(11):1488-91.

[33] Ricci R, Dei Tos AP, Rindi G. On the prevalence of KRAS mutations in GISTs. *Virchows Arch.* 2013; 463(6):847.

[34] Italiano A, Chen CL, Sung YS, et al. SDHA loss of function mutations in a subset of young adult wild-type gastrointestinal stromal tumors. *BMC Cancer* 2012; 12:408.

[35] Dwight T, Benn DE, Clarkson A, et al. Loss of SDHA expression identifies SDHA mutations in succinate dehydrogenase-deficient gastrointestinal stromal tumors. *Am. J. Surg. Pathol.* 2013; 37(2):226-33.

[36] Wagner AJ, Remillard SP, Zhang YX, et al. Loss of expression of SDHA predicts SDHA mutations in gastrointestinal stromal tumors. *Mod. Pathol.* 2013; 26(2):289-94.

[37] Ernst SI, Hubbs AE, Przygodzki RM, et al., KIT mutation portends poor prognosis in gastrointestinal stromal/smooth muscle tumors. *Lab. Invest.* 1998; 78(12):1633-6.

[38] Taniguchi M, Nishida T, Hirota S, et al. Effect of c-kit mutation on prognosis of gastrointestinal stromal tumors. *Cancer Res* 1999; 59(17):4297-300.

[39] Ma YY, Yu S, He XJ, et al. Involvement of c-KIT mutation in the development of gastrointestinal stromal tumors through proliferation promotion and apoptosis inhibition. *Onco Targets Ther* 2014; 7:637-43.

[40] Demetri GD, von Mehren M, Blanke CD, et al. Efficacy and safety of imatinib mesylate in advanced gastrointestinal stromal tumors. *N. Engl. J. Med.* 2002; 347(7):472-80.

[41] Wardelmann E, Losen I, Hans V, et al. Deletion of Trp-557 and Lys-558 in the juxtamembrane domain of the c-kit protooncogene is associated

with metastatic behavior of gastrointestinal stromal tumors. *Int. J. Cancer* 2003; 106(6):887-95.

[42] Debiec-Rychter M, Sciot R, Le Cesne A, et al. KIT mutations and dose selection for imatinib in patients with advanced gastrointestinal stromal tumours. *Eur. J. Cancer* 2006; 42(8):1093-103.

[43] Heinrich MC, Owzar K, Corless CL, et al. Correlation of kinase genotype and clinical outcome in the North American Intergroup Phase III Trial of imatinib mesylate for treatment of advanced gastrointestinal stromal tumor: CALGB 150105 Study by Cancer and Leukemia Group B and Southwest Oncology Group. *J. Clin. Oncol.* 2008; 26(33):5360-7.

[44] Gastrointestinal Stromal Tumor Meta-Analysis Group (MetaGIST). Comparison of two doses of imatinib for the treatment of unresectable or metastatic gastrointestinal stromal tumors: a meta-analysis of 1,640 patients. *J. Clin. Oncol.* 2010; 28(7):1247-53.

[45] Emile J, Brahimi S, Coindre J, et al. Prognostic value of the most frequent mutations in GIST: Results of the French population-based prospective study MolecGIST. *J. Clin. Oncol.* 2010; 28(15s): ASCO meeting abstract:10034.

[46] Antonescu CR, Viale A, Sarran L, et al. Gene expression in gastrointestinal stromal tumors is distinguished by KIT genotype and anatomic site. *Clin. Cancer Res.* 2004; 10(10):3282-90.

[47] Subramanian S, West RB, Corless CL, et al., Gastrointestinal stromal tumors (GISTs) with KIT and PDGFRA mutations have distinct gene expression profiles. *Oncogene* 2004; 23(47):7780-90.

[48] Chen LL, Trent JC, Wu EF, et al. A missense mutation in KIT kinase domain 1 correlates with imatinib resistance in gastrointestinal stromal tumors. *Cancer Res.* 2004; 64(17):5913-9.

[49] Heinrich MC, Maki RG, Corless CL, et al. Primary and secondary kinase genotypes correlate with the biological and clinical activity of sunitinib in imatinib-resistant gastrointestinal stromal tumor. *J. Clin. Oncol.* 2008; 26(33): 5352-9.

[50] Antonescu CR, Besmer P, Guo T, et al. Acquired resistance to imatinib in gastrointestinal stromal tumor occurs through secondary gene mutation. *Clin. Cancer Res.* 2005; 11(11):4182-90.

[51] Heinrich MC, Corless CL, Blanke CD, et al., Molecular correlates of imatinib resistance in gastrointestinal stromal tumors. *J. Clin. Oncol.* 2006; 24(29):4764-74.

[52] Wardelmann E, Merkelbach-Bruse S, Pauls K, et al. Polyclonal evolution of multiple secondary KIT mutations in gastrointestinal

stromal tumors under treatment with imatinib mesylate. *Clin. Cancer Res.* 2006; 12(6):1743-9.

[53] Nishida T, Kanda T, Nishitani A, et al. Secondary mutations in the kinase domain of the KIT gene are predominant in imatinib-resistant gastrointestinal stromal tumor. *Cancer Sci.* 2008; 99(4):799-804.

[54] Lim KH, Huang MJ, Chen LT, et al. Molecular analysis of secondary kinase mutations in imatinib-resistant gastrointestinal stromal tumors. *Med. Oncol.* 2008; 25(2):207-13.

[55] Demetri GD, van Oosterom AT, Garrett CR, et al. Efficacy and safety of sunitinib in patients with advanced gastrointestinal stromal tumour after failure of imatinib: a randomised controlled trial. *Lancet* 2006; 368(9544):1329-38.

[56] Lasota J, Dansonka-Mieszkowska A, Sobin LH, Miettinen M. A great majority of GISTs with PDGFRA mutations represent gastric tumors of low or no malignant potential. *Lab. Invest.* 2004; 84(7):874-83.

[57] Debiec-Rychter M, Lasota J, Sarlomo-Rikala M, Kordek R, Miettinen M. Chromosomal aberrations in malignant gastrointestinal stromal tumors: correlation with c-KIT gene mutation. *Cancer Genet Cytogenet* 2001; 128(1):24-30.

[58] Gunawan B, von Heydebreck A, Sander B, et al. An oncogenetic tree model in gastrointestinal stromal tumours (GISTs) identifies different pathways of cytogenetic evolution with prognostic implications. *J. Pathol.* 2007; 211(4):463-70.

[59] Assämäki R, Sarlomo-Rikala M, Lopez-Guerrero JA, et al. Array comparative genomic hybridization analysis of chromosomal imbalances and their target genes in gastrointestinal stromal tumors. *Genes Chromosomes Cancer*; 2007; 46(6):564-76.

[60] Kinoshita K, Hirota S, Isozaki K et al. Absence of c-kit gene mutations in gastrointestinal stromal tumours from neurofibromatosis type 1 patients. *J. Pathol.* 2004; 202(1):80-5.

[61] Andersson J, Sihto H, Meis-Kindblom JM, et al. NF1-associated gastrointestinal stromal tumors have unique clinical, phenotypic, and genotypic characteristics. *Am. J. Surg. Pathol.* 2005; 29(9):1170-6.

[62] Yantiss RK, Rosenberg AE, Sarran L, Besmer P, Antonescu CR. Multiple gastrointestinal stromal tumors in type I neurofibromatosis: a pathologic and molecular study. *Mod. Pathol.* 2005; 18(4):475-84.

[63] Takazawa Y, Sakurai S, Sakuma Y, et al. Gastrointestinal stromal tumors of neurofibromatosis type I (von Recklinghausen's disease). *Am. J. Surg. Pathol.*, 2005; 29(6):755-63.

[64] Yamamoto H, Tobo T, Nakamori M, et al. Neurofibromatosis type 1-related gastrointestinal stromal tumors: a special reference to loss of heterozygosity at 14q and 22q. *J. Cancer Res. Clin. Oncol.* 2009; 135(6):791-8.
[65] Gaal J, Stratakis CA, Carney JA, et al. SDHB immunohistochemistry: a useful tool in the diagnosis of Carney-Stratakis and Carney triad gastrointestinal stromal tumors. *Mod. Pathol.* 2011; 24(1):147-51.
[66] Matyakhina L, Bei TA, McWhinney SR, et al. Genetics of carney triad: recurrent losses at chromosome 1 but lack of germline mutations in genes associated with paragangliomas and gastrointestinal stromal tumors. *J. Clin. Endocrinol. Metab.* 2007; 92(8):2938-43.
[67] Pasini B, McWhinney SR, Bei T, et al. Clinical and molecular genetics of patients with the Carney-Stratakis syndrome and germline mutations of the genes coding for the succinate dehydrogenase subunits SDHB, SDHC, and SDHD. *Eur. J. Hum. Genet.* 2008; 16(1):79-88.
[68] Nannini M, Biasco G, Astolfi A, Pantaleo MA. An overview on molecular biology of KIT/PDGFRA wild type (WT) gastrointestinal stromal tumours (GIST). *J. Med. Genet.* 2013; 50(10):653-61.

In: Gastrointestinal Stromal Tumors in Adults … ISBN: 978-1-63483-679-1
Editor: Atif A. Ahmed

Chapter 3

IMAGING OF GASTROINTESTINAL STROMAL TUMOURS

Sujata Patnaik*
Department of Radiology and Imageology
Nizam's Institute of Medical Sciences, Punjagutta, Hyderabad, India

ABSTRACT

Gastrointestinal stromal tumour (GIST) is most commonly found in the stomach and small bowel and exhibits distinct radiological features. Imaging studies are useful in determining the exact location and size of the tumour. Smaller size and homogenous attenuation favour a benign lesion. Metastasis at presentation is seen in more than 50% of cases. The liver is the most common site of metastasis followed by peritoneum. However, lung, bone and lymph node metastases are not uncommon. Computed tomography (CT) is the gold standard modality in the initial diagnosis and staging of GIST. Positron emission tomography combined with CT is the investigation of choice for assessment of response by virtue of its unique dynamic functional characteristics.

* Corresponding author: sujata_patnaik222@yahoo.co.in.

NOMENCLATURE

Gastrointestinal stromal tumours (GISTs) are a group of mesenchymal tumours that predominantly exhibit an alternate expression or activation of the oncogene KIT (CD117), which is a tyrosine kinase growth factor receptor. Schaldenbrand and Appleman first used the term GIST in 1984 [1]. These tumours were previously referred as leiomyomas, leiomyosarcomas, leiomyoblastomas or schwannomas. After years of controversies and debates, GISTs are now defined as distinct spindle cell, epithelioid or occasionally pleomorphic mesenchymal tumours of the gastrointestinal tract, which express the KIT protein (CD117, stem cell factor receptor) as detected by immunohistochemistry. They are thought to arise from the interstitial cells of Cajal, which are pluripotent mesenchymal stem cells that act as pacemaker cells controlling gastrointestinal motility [2].

INCIDENCE

Mesenchymal tumours account for only 0.1 to 3% of all gastrointestinal (GI) neoplasms and 5-7% of GI sarcomas [3]. GISTs are the most common mesenchymal neoplasms of the gastrointestinal tract. Incidence in the general population is 10-20 cases per million [4, 5]. Recent studies suggest that incidentally detected sub-centimetre lesions (GIST tumourlets) may be underestimated and these frequently show c-KIT mutations [6].

PRESENTATION

GISTs are subepithelial neoplasms, found anywhere in the gastrointestinal tract from oesophagus to anus; but are mostly located in stomach (60%), small bowel (30%) and elsewhere in GI tract in the rest of cases [7]. Small number, less than 2%, of mesenchymal tumours with similar histopathological characteristics to GIST, have been increasingly described in the omentum, mesentery, retroperitoneum, abdominal wall, gallbladder, pancreas and rectovaginal septum and are called extraintestinal GIST (EGIST) [8]. GISTs account for 1-3% of gastric neoplasms, 20% of small bowel neoplasms and 0.2-1% of colorectal cancer [9]. Sometimes the origin cannot be established because of extensive peritoneal spread. GISTs are multicentric in fewer than

5% of the cases. These tumours occur mostly in middle aged and older patients with no sex predilection. GIST has been reported in all ages including newborns [10]. Paediatric GIST accounts for 1-2% of all GIST [11].

Clinical presentation is variable reflecting variability of radiographic appearance, location and biological behaviour. Approximately 10-30% are asymptomatic. Because of nonspecific clinical symptoms and variable size and exophytic tumour growth, GISTs are often not detected until late in their course or detected incidentally. Symptomatic patients may present with non-specific vague abdominal pain, early satiety, flatulence, fever, night-sweats, anaemia, nausea and vomiting or gastrointestinal bleeding (due to mucosal ulceration) [12]. Oesophageal GIST may present with dysphagia, cough, bleeding or as an incidental posterior mediastinal mass [13]. A large tumour with profound symptoms is expected to be aggressive with local spread and metastasis.

CHOICE OF IMAGING MODALITIES

All types of imaging modalities can be used, depending on the tumour location and size. Plain radiographs reveal large soft tissue mass displacing bowel loops or causing mediastinal widening (Figure 1). Barium study reveals polypoidal mass seen as filling defect with right / obtuse angle with bowel lumen (Figure 1, 2). Those protruding into the lumen produce acute angle while exophytic ones produce obtuse angle. Although ultrasound is an initial investigational modality, often a tumour at presentation reaches such a large size that the site of origin cannot be identified. Large tumours are complex-looking with cystic and solid components. Liver metastasis can be easily picked up by ultrasonography. Endoscopic ultrasound is used for tumours less than 2 cm detected by endoscopy. A high frequency probe delineates bowel wall layer by layer and can locate site of origin and tumour vascularity (Figure 1). Endoscopic ultrasound is useful for visualising tumours in the oesophagus, stomach, duodenum and rectum. Ultrasound guidance is also helpful for biopsy. However such biopsy is not usually recommended due to risk of peritoneal seedling or tumour dehiscence of necrotic debris [14]. Computed tomography (CT) is the modality of choice, not only for the diagnosis but also for staging and to assess tumour response. Oral and IV contrast should be used to define the bowel margins [15]. Tumour vascularity can be visualised in axial images and in reconstructed images by multi-slice CT (Figure 3, 4).

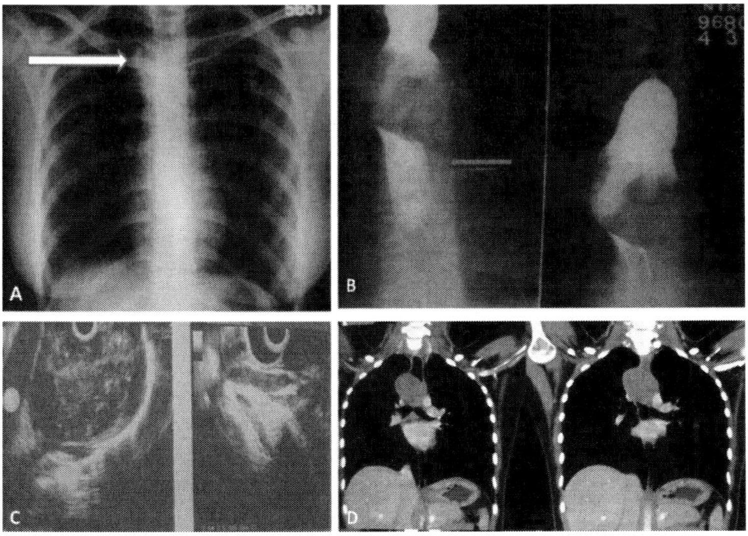

Figure 1. Oesophageal GIST in 24 year female patient.
A. Chest radiograph revealing mediastinal widening (white arrow)
B. Arrow showing smooth filling defect with obtuse angle with the lumen in barium swallow
C & D. Mass appears homogenously isoechoic in ultrasonography and isodense in endoluminal ultrasound and CT scan.

Due to the high soft-tissue contrast and multi-planar capabilities, the origin of the tumour and its relation to adjacent tissues and major vessels can be well studied in magnetic resonance imaging (MRI) which is accepted as superior to CT in this aspect and is increasingly used. MRI is also superior to CT in studying hepatic metastasis and rectal GIST. It has limited sensitivity for detection of peritoneal deposits. MRI can differentiate high density tumour from haemorrhage. In a recent study, Yu MH et al. observed that the tumours with intramural cystic change and low apparent diffusion coefficient (ADC) value on MRI predicted high malignant potential of a GIST (16,17). Dynamic MRI is excellent for tumour viability and quantitative status of angiogenesis. *Diffusion weighted imaging* (DWI) is unable to differentiate low and high grade GIST.

Positron emission tomography (PET) scan is not an initial modality for diagnosis due to its lack of specificity; but useful for detecting an unknown primary site or for solving confusion about a doubtful lesion on CT. The reported sensitivity of PET scan for GIST detection is 86 to 100% [18]. Fluorodeoxyglucose-Positron emission tomography (FDG PET) helps to differentiate pseudo-progression (an increase in size due to myxoid degeneration or intra tumoral bleed) from true progression. It is also helpful for metastatic evaluation in a biopsy proven malignancy and to monitor therapy and also helpful in short-term follow up of marginally resected GIST [19].

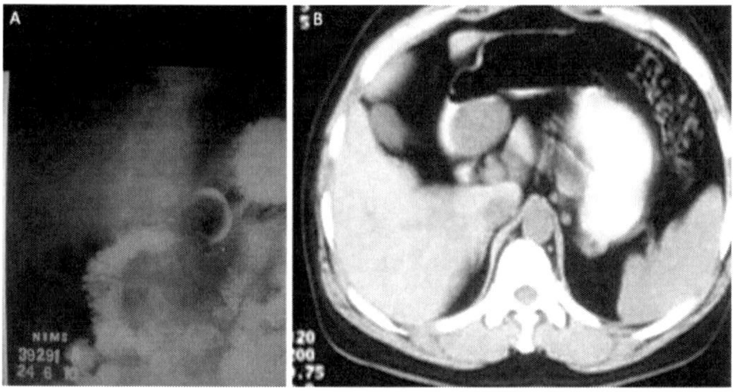

Figure 2. Gastric GIST in 46-year male patient. A. Polypoidal filling defect with smooth contour in barium meal examination. B. NECT axial scan depicting the lesion.

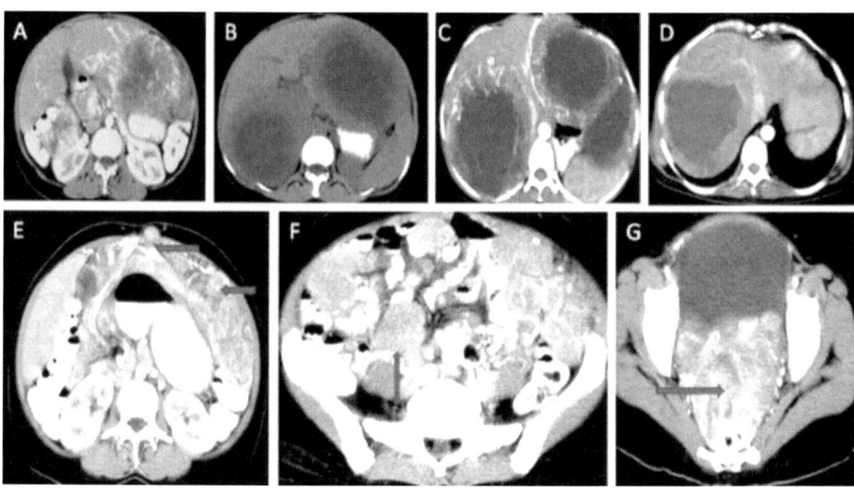

Figure 3. Jejunal GIST in 32 year female patient. A. Axial contrast enhanced CT showing extensive neovascularity in Jejunal space-occupying lesion. B, C, D. The liver metastases in plain (B), contrast enhanced images in arterial (C), delayed (D) images revealing vascularity and enhancement. E, F, G. Extensive omental, subcutaneous deposits (E), mesenteric deposits (F), in pouch of Douglas displacing rectum posteriorly (G) indicated by arrow.

Angiography may be done as part of investigation when there is bleeding. Prominent internal arterial and venous branching pattern will be displayed together with evidence of extravasations. Prominent feeding artery and draining vein as well as tumour staining with contrast will also be highlighted. Similar characteristics are also observed in metastases. Demonstration of vascular suply may also aid in route mapping prior to surgery [20]. Increased recognition of GIST and prolonged survival made imaging increasingly important not only for diagnosis but also for monitoring effects of chemotherapy and detecting tumour progression. Moreover early detection and surgery may improve the prognosis of patients.

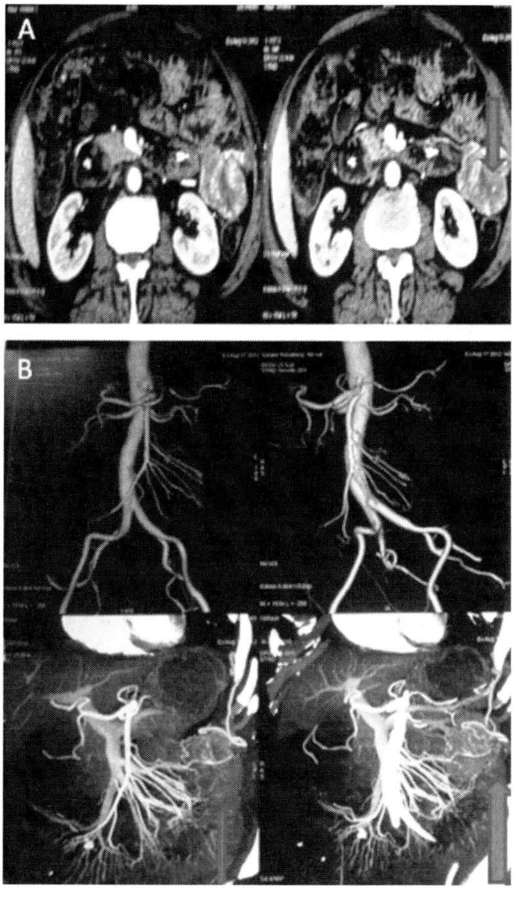

Figure 4. A and B. Small bowel GIST in a middle aged male demonstrated in contrast enhanced CT in axial image and vascular supply in coronal MPR indicated by arrow.

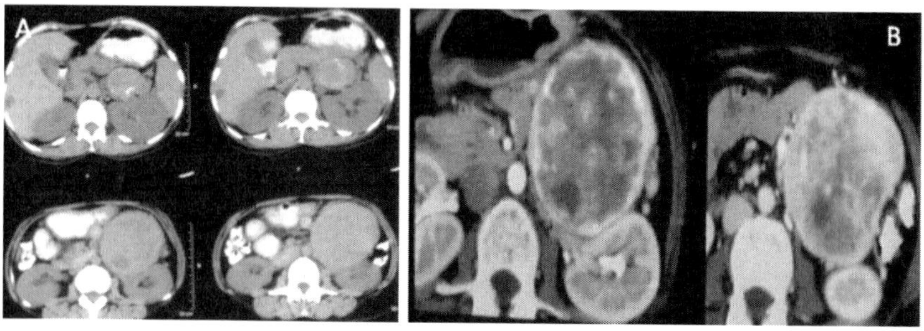

Figure 8. Retroperitoneal GIST in a 39-year old male patient. A and B. Calcification and moderate inhomogeneous enhancement in retroperitoneal GIST, features similar to gastric GIST.

Smaller lesions are homogenous to begin with but, as they grow larger they may become heterogeneous. Large tumours can outstrip their blood supply leading to necrosis, cavitation and communication with lumen. Hence internal air, calcification, haemorrhage, and/or fluid level may be noted (Figure 8, 9). It is observed that tumours larger than 6 cm show central necrosis, whereas in tumour of 3 cm or less do not. Mucosal ulceration is seen in luminal surface of tumours in up to 50% cases. Haemorrhage with hemoperitoneum was observed in one of our cases, which was a high risk gastric GIST (Figure 5,10). Presence of air due to fistulisation is characteristic of GIST and is seldom observed in other malignancies [21]. Since tumours are hypervascular, neovascularity may be seen in contrast enhanced scans (Figure 3,4). Often the mass displaces adjacent organs or vessels. It is important to observe the contour. Ill-defined margins, mesenteric infiltration and local invasion to adjacent structures indicate malignant nature. Similar to lymphoma, enteric GIST may show aneurismal dilatation of the bowel in 33% of cases [22]. This may be due to cavitary nature of this fast growing tumour that allows enlargement of lumen. The tumour may damage the myenteric plexus allowing dilatation of lumen (Figure 11). Ascites is rare in GIST, as they do not incite inflammatory response. Ascites may develop following therapy or can occur due to perforation, rupture or bleeding in GIST (Figure 5, 10) [23].

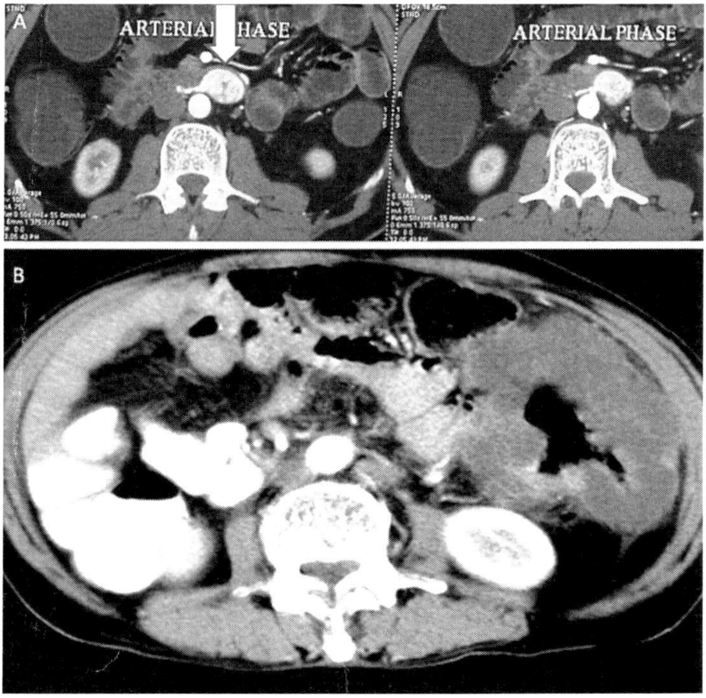

Figure 9. Duodenal and Jejunal GIST in 45-year old and 69-year old male patients. A, B. Intraluminal homogenously enhancing duodenal and heterogeneously enhancing exophytic Jejunal GISTS.

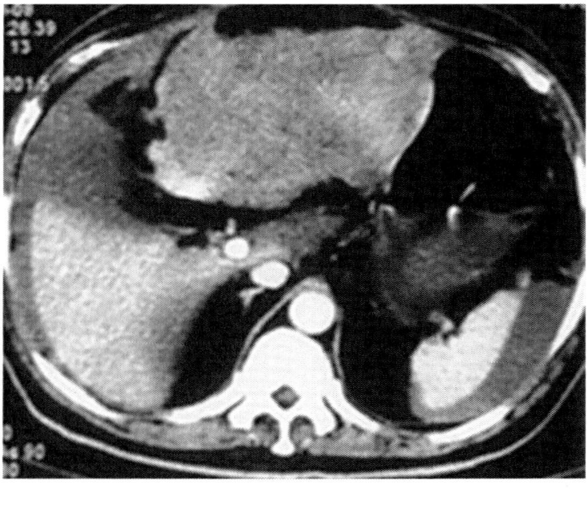

Figure 10. Gastric GIST with hemoperitoneum in a 70 years old male patient.

SITE SPECIFIC FEATURES

Oesophageal GIST

The oesophagus is a relatively uncommon site for GIST where leiomyoma dominates and accounts for 75% of mesenchymal tumours; whereas in the stomach, small bowel, colon, and anorectum almost all mesenchymal tumours are GIST. These tumours usually occur in the distal third of oesophagus and can measure up to 25 cm in size [13]. Chest radiographs reveal soft tissue mass in mediastinum or soft tissue mass distorting the gastric bubble. Barium studies reveal smooth intramural mass or large ulcerated mass extending to oesophageal lumen (Figure 1). On computerized tomography, these lesions may be homogenous or heterogeneous in attenuation due to central areas of necrosis, haemorrhage or cystic degeneration [24]. Benign entities to consider in the differential of GIST in this location include leiomyoma, duplication cyst, lipoma, and hemangioma. When the lesion is submucosal, endoluminal ultrasound guided fine needle aspiration cytology (FNAC) is a good technique for final diagnosis. An intraluminal polypoidal GIST has to be differentiated from papilloma, adenoma, inflammatory polyp, fibrovascular polyp and carcinoma [25]. In contrast to leiomyomas, GISTs tend to be distal, larger and more heterogeneous and enhancing on CT and are FDG avid on PET [25]. In advanced stages when there is extension to mediastinum, GISTs are to be differentiated from carcinoma, lymphoma, melanoma and leiomyosarcoma (Figure 12).

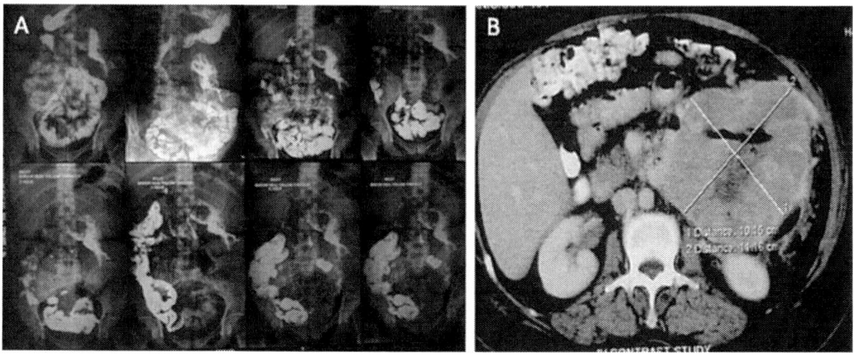

Figure 11. Small bowel GIST in 45 years old female patient. A&B. Barium study showing large ulceration indicated by arrow and same depicted in figure B with aneurysmal dilatation of lumen.

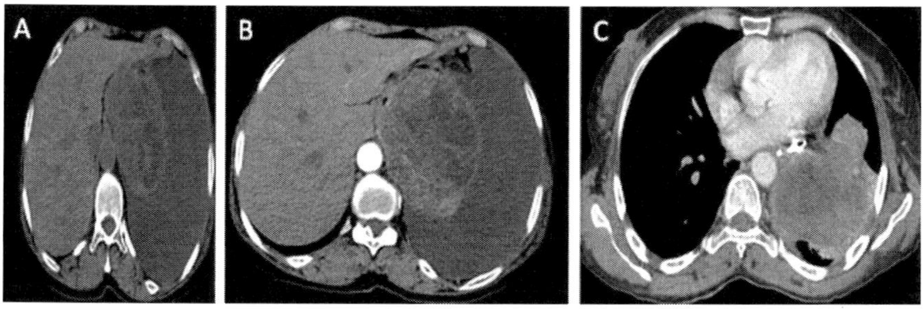

Figure 12. Oesophageal GIST. A, B &C. Exophytic growth in plain and contrast enhanced scan revealing inhomogeneous enhancement and mimicking carcinoma in A&B. On treatment there is reduction in size of mass (C).

Gastric GIST

The stomach is the most frequent location for GIST and constitutes 2-3% of all gastric tumours. Benign GISTs are three times more common than malignant tumours and appear as non-specific soft tissue mass indenting or displacing the gastric air shadow in plain radiographs. Rarely calcifications may occur and be visible in radiographs. Collection of abnormal air may be appreciated in necrotic tumours (Figure 6). In barium studies, submucosal GIST have non-specific features of any submucosal tumour similar to leiomyoma or leiomyosarcoma. The tumour size may range from 4-25 cm. The margin of the tumour lesion may form obtuse or right angle with the wall. When viewed on profile it is smoothly circumscribed, and the non-ulcerated mucosal surface of the mass appears smooth. When ulcerated, the lesion appears as bull's-eye or target-like. In case of tumour necrosis and cavitation, the barium may fill the inner part of the necrotic tumour. Sometimes a focal polypoidal mass may appear as smooth filling defect (Figure 2) [26].

CT reliably demonstrates the site, size, contour and spread of the tumour. The tumour pedicle may rarely be demonstrated. Careful evaluation of the wall may reveal subtle thickening that helps to establish the stomach as the origin of mass. The origin may sometimes be difficult to appreciate when the mass is large. Large tumours have extensive haemorrhage and necrosis in the form of large cystic spaces and cavities. Cavities may communicate with the gastric lumen and contain air, air- fluid level, and/or oral contrast [27]. Calcification is rarely seen. A peripheral enhancement with neovascularity is seen in the majority of cases (Figure 6, 13, 14) [28]. Homogenous enhancement is seen in only a minority of cases. Vascular supply and the course of the pedicle can be demonstrated with CT angiography. Extra-gastric spread to the omentum, liver and peritoneum is seen in 86% of cases [23].

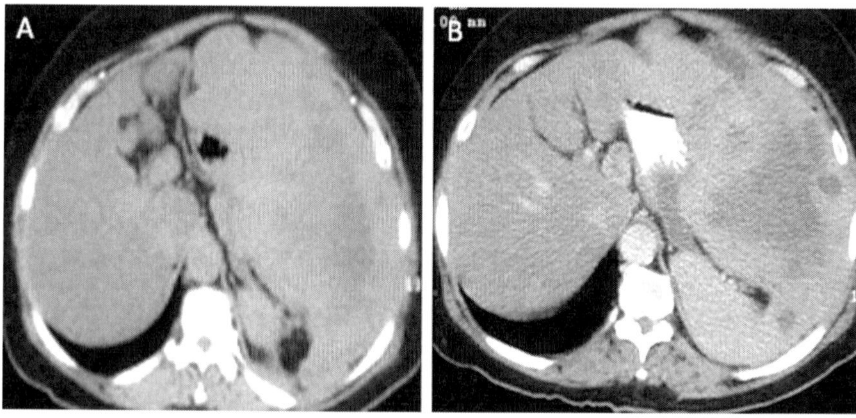

Figure 13. A, B: Large exophytic growth with ill-defined pedicle in gastric GIST in a 51-year old male.

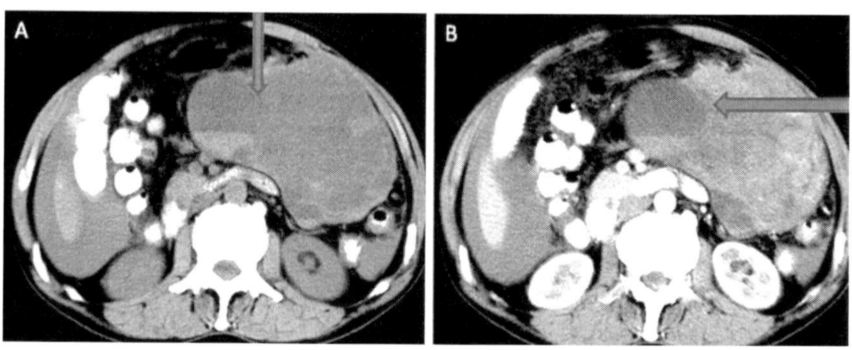

Figure 14. Gastric GIST 50 year old male. A, B. Plain and contrast enhanced scans demonstrating fluid level.

MRI features are variable and depends on the degree of necrosis and haemorrhage. The solid portion of the tumour is typically low in T1W, yields a high signal in T2W images and enhances on contrast. MRI is sometimes helpful to detect the site of origin when it is doubtful on CT scan and can delineate the tumour relationship to adjacent organs and major blood vessels. Tumour perforation is uncommon, occurs up to 20% cases and can cause hemoperitoneum or peritonitis (Figure 5). A differential diagnosis of adenocarcinoma or lymphoma is entertained when the large exophytic component is not seen. Moreover, local lymphadenopathy or extensive adenopathy is not typically seen in adult GIST.

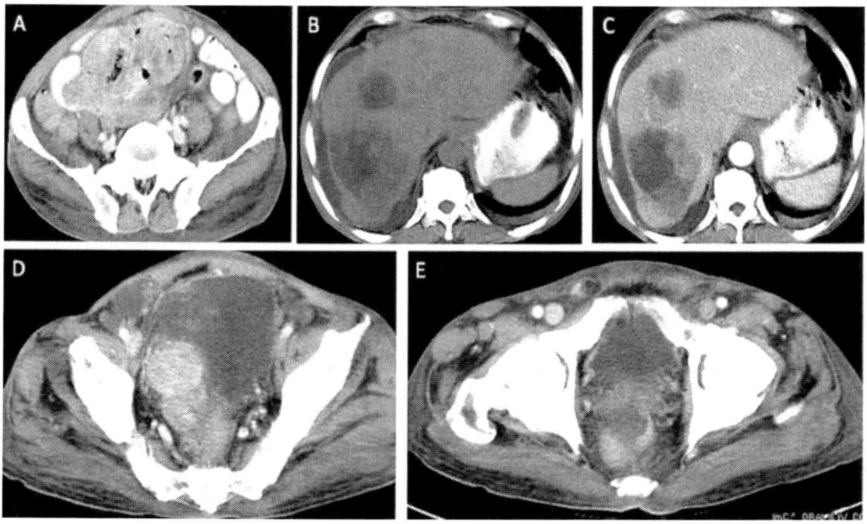

Figure 15. GIST of terminal ileum in a 60 year old male. A. Mass in terminal ileum encasing adjacent bowel loops. B, C, D, E: multiple liver, peritoneal, pelvis and pouch of Douglas deposits.

Small Bowel GIST

GIST in the small intestine may have a more malignant course compared with gastric GIST of the same size. Plain radiographs may reveal small bowel dilatation if there is obstruction, soft tissue mass or abnormal air in cases of fistulisation (Figure 11). Barium studies may show intraluminal mass and mucosal ulceration, if sub-mucosal. There can be extra-serosal growth with mass effect on adjacent bowel segments. Intra-luminal, mural, and extra-serosal masses can be seen in CT (Figure 9). CT and MRI depict the same features as gastric GIST. Extension to adjacent bowel, encasement of colon, bladder, ureter and abdominal wall and metastasis to liver, omentum and peritoneum can all be well seen on CT (Figure 15). Aneurysmal dilatation may be seen. This is partially because of the cavitary nature of fast growing tumours allowing enlargement of the apparent lumen (Figures 11). The tumour may damage the myenteric plexus allowing dilatation of the lumen. Cavitation may allow air to collect in non-dependent portions of large tumours, described as the *Torricelli –Bernousilli crescentic* necrosis sign (Figures 11). Intussusception may be seen in benign small bowel GIST. Differential diagnoses to be considered include adenocarcinoma, lymphoma and metastases. On MR, GISTs show variable enhancement with areas of necrosis. Important entities that need to be differentiated on MR include adenocarcinoma, lymphoma, mesenteric fibromatosis (desmoid tumour), inflammatory pseudo-tumour, sclerosing mesenteritis and metastatic disease [23].

Colonic GIST

Primary colonic involvement is less common accounting for 5% of all GIST. Tumour size varies from 8 -18 cm. The appearance is radiologically similar to gastric GIST. The mass is transmural with central areas of haemorrhage, cystic change, necrosis, and calcifications showing heterogeneous enhancement, and sometimes has circumferential growth and aneurismal dilatation. It can closely mimic leiomyosarcoma (Figure 16). When small and confined, they may be well seen on barium studies. The differential diagnosis includes adenocarcinoma, lymphoma, metastases, leiomyosarcoma and retroperitoneal sarcomas [13, 29].

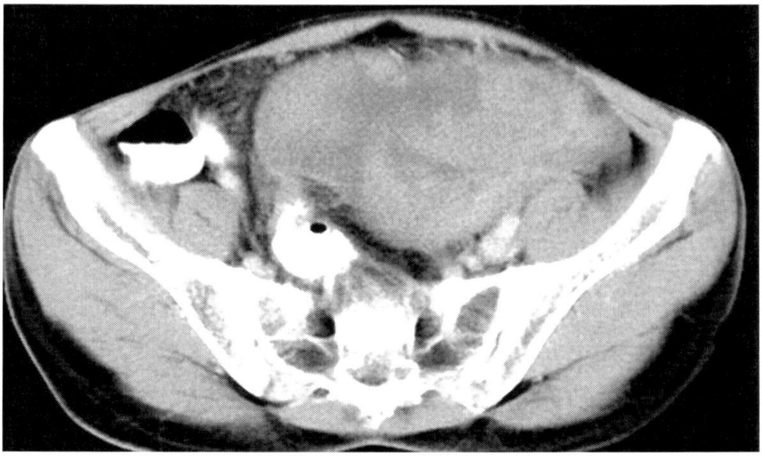

Figure 16. Sigmoid GIST in a 45 year old male patient.

Anorectal GIST

GISTs in this location are most commonly mural and expand the rectal wall. Therefore, a focal well circumscribed mural mass is the most common finding in CT which generally exhibits features similar to GIST in other locations (Figure 17). Mucosal ulceration may be present. A focal intraluminal filling defect is one of the least common appearances. Local spread may occur to ischeo-rectal fossa, vagina and prostate (Figure 17) [30]. On MRI, T1 weighted images have uniform intermediate intensity signals and on T2 a heterogeneous high signal intensity, with heterogeneous enhancement on contrast [31]. Both epithelial and non-epithelial neoplasms of the region need to be differentiated. Rectal adenocarcinoma, carcinoid, leiomyoma, leiomyosarcoma, prostatic adenocarcimoma and sarcoma can be confused with GIST (23).

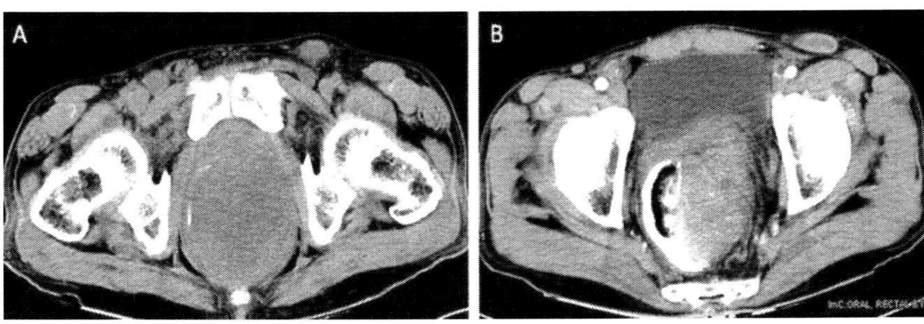

Figure 17. A,B: Rectal GIST in a 64 year old male patient with large exophytic growth from rectum infiltrating prostate, seminal vesicle locally and lymph node metastasis as indicated by arrow.

GIST in the Mesentery and Omentum

EGIST have predilection for mesentery in 22.2-42.9% of cases, for the omentum in 25-28.6%, and the retroperitoneum in 10.7-33.3% [8, 32]. The median size of primary omental/mesenteric GIST was 16.5 cm in the series reported by Miettinen et al. [33]. The appearance may be complex on cross sectional imaging due to haemorrhage and necrosis. The cystic component of mass predominates and peripheral solid portions show enhancement (Figure 18). Sometimes, the origin of GIST cannot be established because of extensive peritoneal metastasis and tumours are confused with peritoneal carcinomatosis (Figure 19), lymphomatosis, and leiomyomatosis peritonealis disseminata.

Imaging features of single large mesenteric /omental GIST may mimic leiomyosarcoma, malignant fibrous histiocytoma, fibrosarcoma, liposarcoma. Metastatic GIST to omentum and mesentery is typically in the form of multiple masses throughout the peritoneal cavity when they are confused with peritoneal carcinomatosis, lymphomatosis or leiomyomatosis peritonealis disseminate (Figure 20) [34].

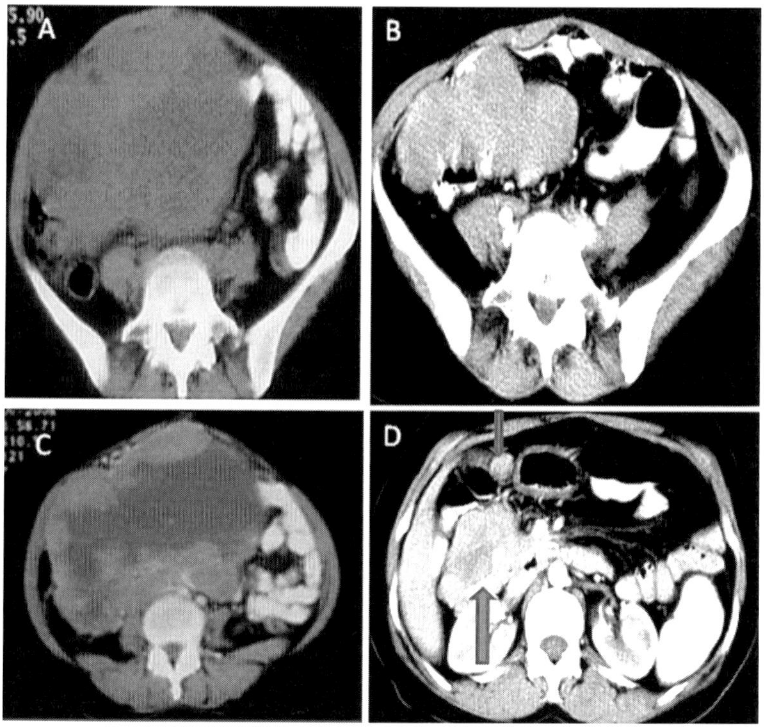

Figure 18. mesenteric GIST in a 50 year old female patient. A,C. Mesenteric GIST has similar characteristics as gastric GIST. B, D. Post-operative recurrence with peritoneal deposits indicated by arrow.

GIST in the Retroperitoneum

EGIST arising from retroperitoneum is extremely rare. Preoperative diagnosis is very difficult and patients often undergo surgery for the diagnosis of any suspicious abdominal mass. Histologically and immunohistochemically they are similar to GIST in other locations. However, the clinical and prognostic factors are not yet defined. On imaging, small tumours appear homogenous and well defined. Large tumours are heterogeneous and ill-defined with necrosis, haemorrhage, cavitation, calcification, invasion and hepatic metastases (Figure 8, 21) [15]. When the size is more than 10 cm, the chances of malignancy are high. Other differentials include malignant fibrous histiocytoma, lipo-or fibrosarcoma and leiomyosarcoma. Cure is possible if complete en bloc removal of the mass with contiguous tissue and lymph nodes can be achieved.

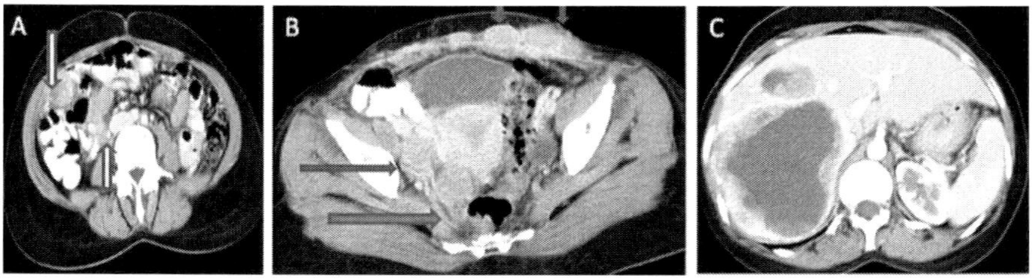

Figure 19. GISTS of unknown origin (30f). A. Peritoneal masses. B. Pelvic deposits and subcutaneous deposits. C. Liver metastases.

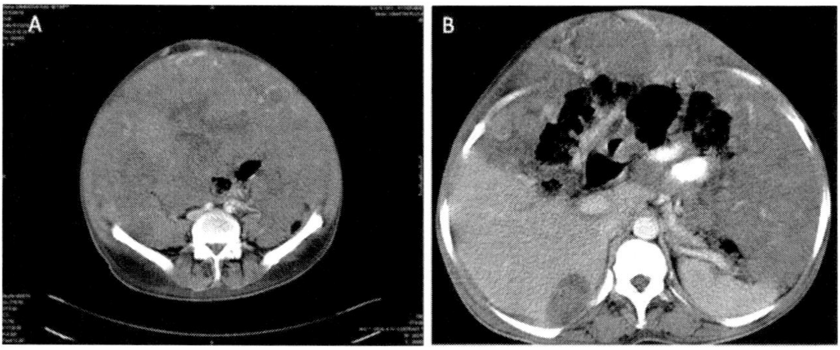

Figure 20. A, B. Extensive peritoneal, mesenteric, omental deposits and scalloping of liver (45m).

FAMILIAL GIST AND ASSOCIATION WITH SYNDROMES

Recently GISTs have been increasingly documented as abdominal manifestation of neurofibromatosis type 1 (NF1). GISTs are detected in 25% of NF1 patients at autopsy [35]. Multicentric GISTs are associated with NF1 and familial GIST and are seen in less than 5%. Patients with NF1 often have multiple small intestinal GISTs (Figure 22) [36]. GIST is also a feature of Carney's triad which is a rare condition referring to the association of GIST with paraganglioma and pulmonary chondroma [37]. Patients with KIT germ line mutations have an increased prevalence of GIST and other GI autonomic tumours in families [38]. Rare association of Crohn's disease in the terminal ileum with high risk GISTs has been reported [39]. GIST in a 12-year old child was reported in association with neuroblastoma [40].

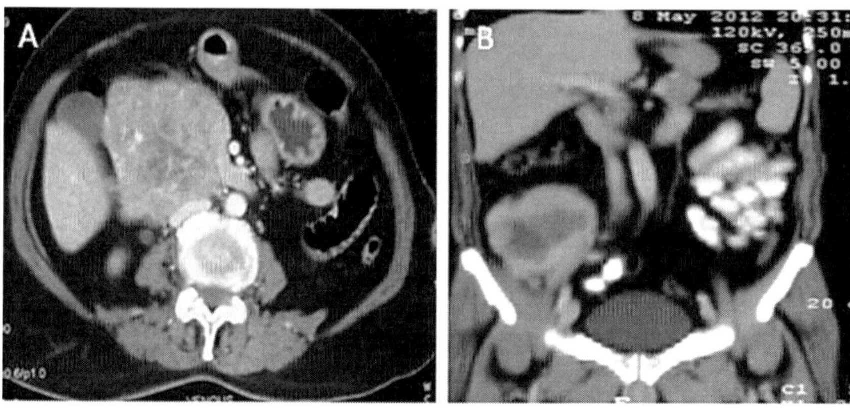

Figure 21. Retroperitoneal GIST. A, B. Retroperitoneal masses in a 72-year old female and 61-year old male patients.

Benign vs Malignant

Benign GISTs outnumber malignant ones in the stomach. Malignant GISTs are more common in the small bowel. Tumours of similar sizes, when located in the small bowel show more malignancy compared to gastric tumours. Most of the oesophageal, colonic and anorectal GISTs are malignant. Tumour size, site and mitosis are three important prognostic factors in GIST. In general malignant tumours are larger, more cellular and show high mitotic activity. A tumour with size more than 6 cm is potentially malignant. Intermediate and low risk GISTs appear radiologically more homogeneous whereas high risk tumours are heterogeneous (Figure 18, 23) [41]. According to DeMatteo et al., all GISTs regardless of size and location have the potential to be malignant. They may recur in the same location or metastasize (Figure

24). Indistinct margins, tissue invasion and peritoneal dissemination are features supporting poor prognosis [3].

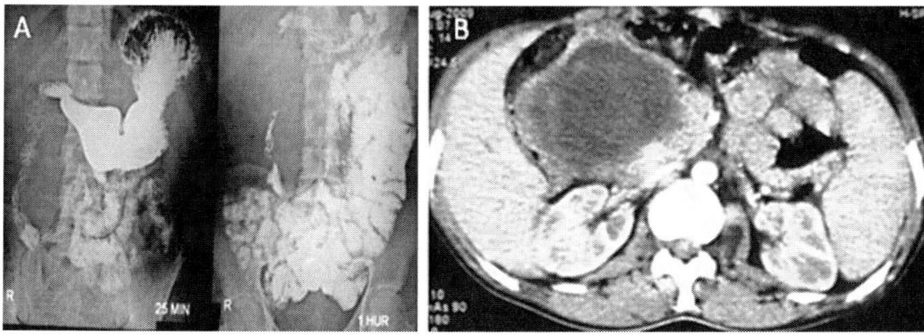

Figure 22. Duodenal GIST with NF1 in a 31 year male. A Barium study showing wide C loop and irregularity of wall, B. Homogenously enhancing mass from duodenum.

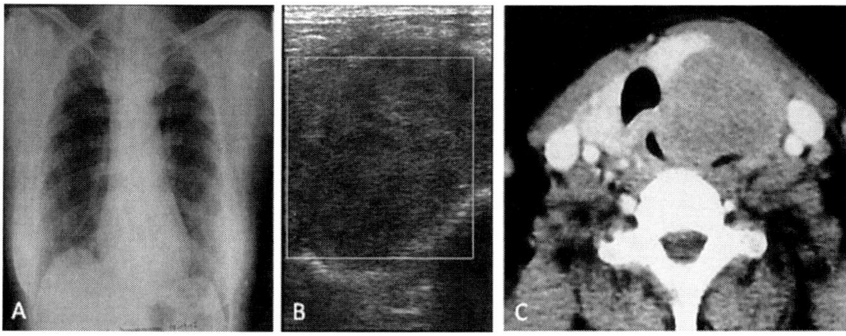

Figure 23. Low grade GIST of oesophagus in a 50-year old female. A. Chest radiograph revealing mediastinal widening. B. Mass is homogenously isoechoic with minimal vascularity. C. On CT scan, the mass is homogenously isodense suggestive of low grade tumour.

METASTASIS

Metastasis at presentation is seen in 50% of cases. Tumours that have metastasis at presentation have very poor prognosis. Metastases to the liver and peritoneum are the most common. Liver is the most common site of metastasis both at presentation and at disease relapse. Metastasis to the lung, lymph nodes or bone are uncommon (Figure 17,26) [42]. GIST rarely spreads to regional lymph nodes (<10%). Local recurrence or metastasis on follow up is a common feature of GIST. In our own study of 42 cases, 52.3% showed metastasis on presentation. The mesentery, omentum and liver were the most frequent sites for metastasis. Due to the longer survival of patients, metastases are also seen in other sites such as the lung and lymph nodes, where they were thought to be rare. Metastatic tumours have attenuation and enhancement characteristics similar to the primary tumours and often reveal necrosis, haemorrhage and calcification [43].

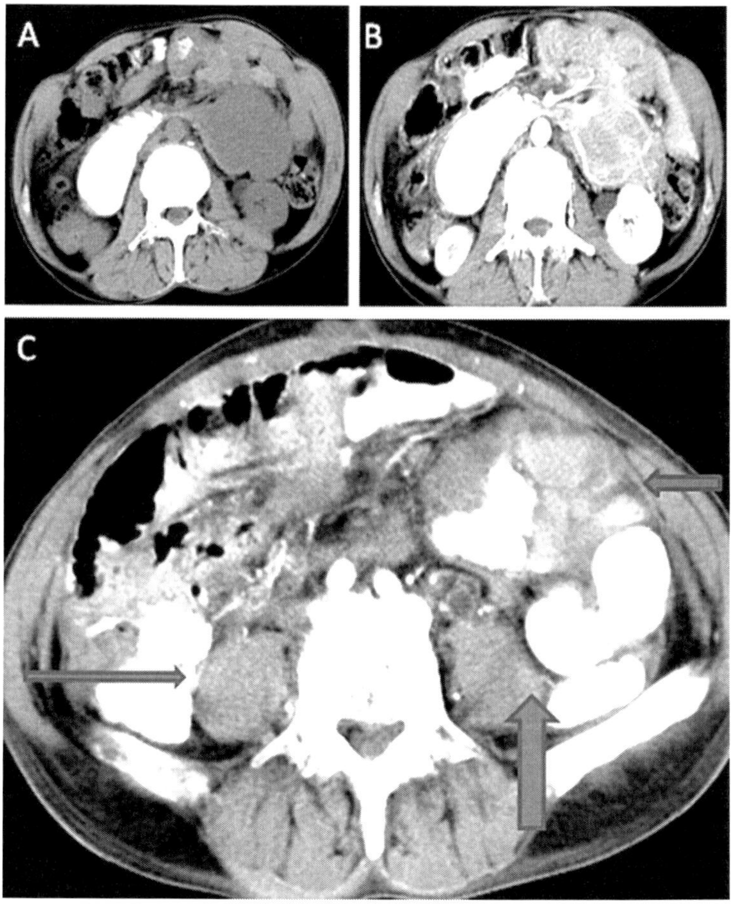

Figure 24. Jejunal GIST in a 35-year male patient. A, B, C. Despite the small size of the tumor, there was post-operative recurrence with extensive peritoneal deposits (Figure -24C).

CT of metastatic tumours is likely to be heterogeneous with central necrosis and peripheral enhancement. Visceral obstruction is rare feature. Ascites is unusual. Hepatic metastases are usually multiple, may involve both lobes and are due to spread via the portal vein. In pre-contrast scans, the lesions appear hypodense or isodense to the liver except when there is retained haemorrhage, proteinaceous material, or calcification. Haemorrhage can occur in metastasis as well (Figure 25). Low attenuation at the centre often indicates necrosis of solid areas that may become cystic. Cystic components may be heterogeneous and marked by irregular and variable solid periphery (Figure 3). Lesions enhance in late arterial or portal venous phase (Figure 26). Cystic metastatic tumours are rare and may have fluid- fluid level and multicystic appearance. Lesions usually become smaller and more cystic after treatment (Figure 27) [44]. Multi-cystic tumours may appear like simple cysts; the density differentiates them from one another. Similar cystic changes also occur in mesenteric and peritoneal deposits after chemotherapy.

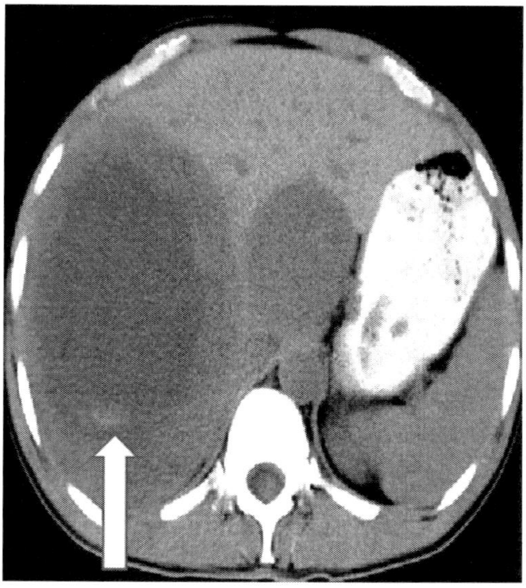

Figure 25. Small bowel GIST with liver metastasis showing bleed in a 42-year old male patient.

Mesenteric/omental tumour deposits are either due to surgery or spread of primary tumour. Metastatic masses present low density at the centre and show heterogeneous enhancement. Lesions appear as large discrete masses or multiple nodules involving the peritoneal surface and subperitoneal spaces

(Figure 3, 15, 19). Less commonly, they reveal diffuse hypervascular omental /peritoneal caking (Figure 20). Sometimes it is difficult to differentiate tumours from un-opacified bowel when they grow around vessels and encase them without thrombosis. Because of mobility of the omentum, some masses appear in different positions on subsequent scans. Despite the presence of large tumour masses in the mesentery/omentum, ascites is rare. Peritoneal carcinomatosis and lymphoma can be close mimics [45].

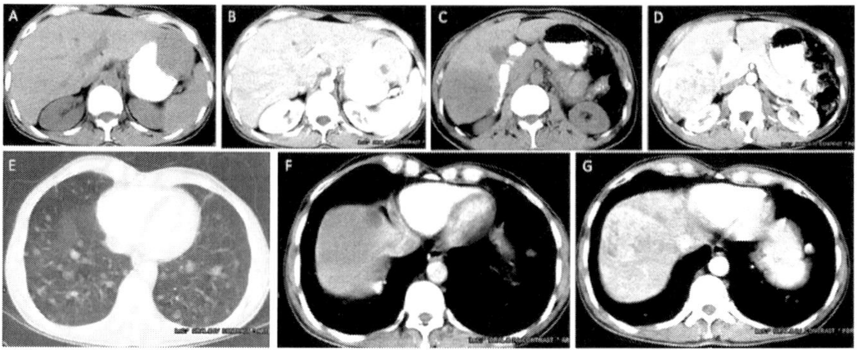

Figure 26. Gastric GIST in a 61-year old male patient. A, B. Primary mass. C, D. Enhancing liver metastases. E. Multiple pulmonary nodules in both lungs in lung window. F, G. In mediastinal window, nodule shows enhancement.

Bone metastases are rare. The spine and pelvis are common sites. Skull involvement is rare and reported in few cases. They appear lytic, well defined and often multiple in the axial skeleton. Extra osseous soft tissue component is observed. CT of bone metastasis is not specific and imaging characteristics are similar to the primary mass (Figure 28). FDG-PET shows high uptake. Half of the bone metastasis cases respond to treatment and develop sclerotic margins.

Less commonly, metastases are found in soft tissue, lung, and pleura. The incidence of lung metastases is increasing due to long survival of patients. Lung lesions initially are micro-nodules without clinical significance. Radiologically they appear as well defined nodules and hyperdense without central necrosis on IV contrast studies (Figure 26). GIST lung metastases have low biologic aggressiveness compared to primary tumours or metastases at other sites. Lung metastases respond differently to treatment unlike liver or peritoneal deposits. Cutaneous deposits are rare and are probably due to spread through abdominal scars and they appear similar to the primary mass (Figures 3, 19) [46].

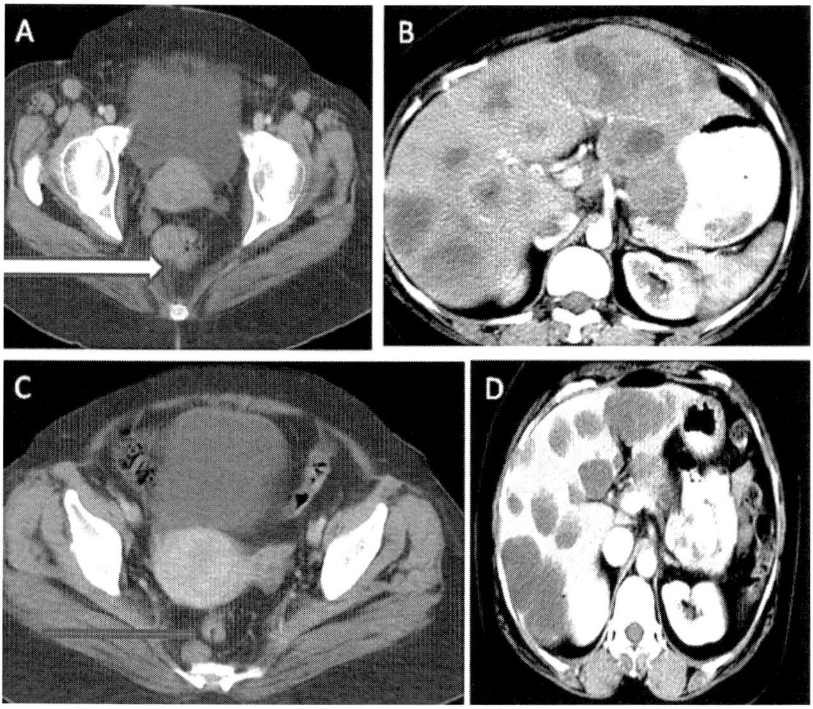

Figure 27. Rectal GIST in 45-year old female patient. A, B. Pre-treatment mass in rectum and liver metastases. C, D. Resolution of the primary mass on follow up; Liver lesions are more cystic and there is a new appearance of pelvic deposits.

GIST metastasis to lymph nodes is rare. It is hypothesized that when tumour cells invade liver, they tend to spread to the peripheral blood and migrate to lymph nodes. Metastatic tumour in nodes appears similar to the primary mass in attenuation and enhancement pattern and sometime it may be hyper-echoic (Figure 17). When there is lymphadenopathy, one has to think of an alternate diagnosis.

PEDIATRIC GIST

Though GIST occur predominantly after age of 50, five to 25% occur in patients less than 40 yrs and less than 3% occur in children [47]. Paediatric GIST typically occurs more frequently in females in contrast to adult GIST and more often in association with familial disorders such as neurofibromatosis-1 (NF1), the Carney triad and Carney-Stratakis syndrome [10, 48]. Most of them also lack mutations in *KIT* and *PDGFRA*. Carney-Stratakis syndrome refers to occurrence of GIST and paraganglioma in children with inherited germline mutations of *SDH* in the absence of *KIT* or *PDGFRA* mutations. About 12% have germline mutations in a gene that codes for a sub-unit of the SDH enzyme with loss of function [49].

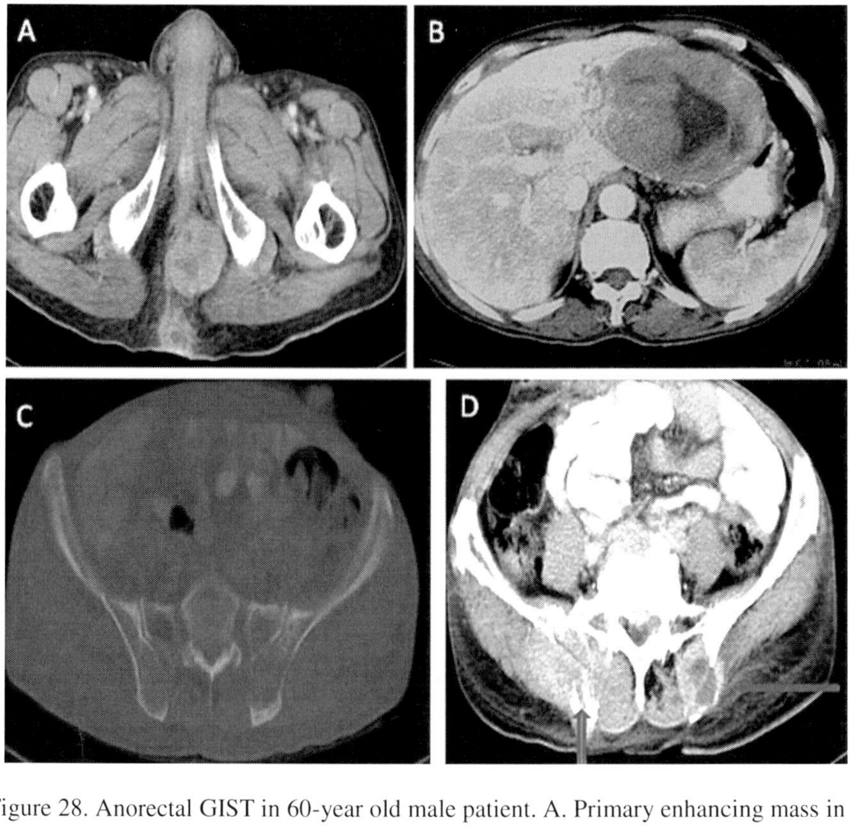

Figure 28. Anorectal GIST in 60-year old male patient. A. Primary enhancing mass in rectum. B. Liver metastasis. C, D. Bone metastasis in bone window and soft tissue window showing enhancing soft tissue component along with the lytic lesion.

Chronic GI bleeding, multifocal tumours and lymph node metastasis are more likely in Paediatric GIST. These GISTs are preferentially located in the stomach as multiple nodules and histologically appear epithelioid, or mixed spindle/epithelioid morphology. The recurrence rate in post gastrectomy is high, possibly due to multiplicity of lesions. It is difficult to evaluate clinical outcome due to limited studies. Tumours appear as hypoechoic masses on

USG and it may sometimes be difficult to identify the organ of origin. On CT scan, tumours are well defined in the gastric wall as they show enhancement. MRI appears hypo/isointense to the gastric wall in T2W images. FDG-PET shows the primary mass and metastasis in the lymph nodes [50].

Evaluation of Response to Treatment

Regular follow up is best done with CT/FDG PET. Response is seen as early as one week after treatment. The heterogeneous tumour mass becomes hypo-attenuating and cystic after treatment. Tumor vessels decrease regardless of the size (Figure 27). Tumour size also reduces with treatment. A ten percent decrease in one-dimensional tumour size or 50% decrease in tumor density determined by CT attenuation coefficient in Hounsfield units (HU) indicates a good response. Presence of new nodules within the tumour showing uniform enhancement or ring like enhancement indicates disease progression. The use of perfusion CT in response evaluation is still under investigation. Recurrence of tumour is defined as new focal area of contrast enhancement on CT or MR images and/or hyperintensity signal on T2W MRI and with nodular or irregular thickening of boundaries of treated area (Figure 24) [51]. Development of enhancing tumour nodule within hypo-attenuating lesion regardless of tumour size and development of new metastasis also indicate disease progression.

Conclusion

Radiologic assessment is a valuable step in the management of patients with GIST tumours. All types of imaging modalities can be used based on tumour location and size. Imaging studies are indicated in the initial evaluation of the tumor, judging response to treatment and documenting presence or absence of metastasis and are useful in the follow-up of patients.

REFERENCES

[1] Roberts, PJ; Eisenberg, B. Clinical presentation of gastrointestinal Stromal tumours and treatment of operable disease. *Euro J Cancer*, 2002, 38(supl-5), S37-S38.

[2] Fletcher, CD; Berman, JJ; Corless, C; et al. Diagnosis of gastrointestinal stromal tumors: a consensus approach. *Hum Pathol*, 2002, 33, 459-465.

[3] DeMatteo, RP; Lewis, JJ; Leung, D; Mudan, SS; Woodruff, JM; Brennan, MF. Two hundred Gastrointestinal stromal tumors; recurrence patterns and prognostic factors for survival. *Ann Surgery*, 2000, 231, 51-58.

[4] Miettinen, M; Sarlomo-Rikala, M; Sobin, LH; Lasota, J. Gastrointestinal stromal tumours and leiomyosarcomas in colon: a clinicopathologic, immunohistochemical and molecular genetic study of 44 cases. *Am J Surg Pathol*, 2000, 24, 1339-1352.

[5] Miettinen, M; El-Rifai, WHL; Sobin, L; Lasota, J. Evaluation of malignancy and prognosis of gastrointestinal stromal tumors: a review. *Hum Pathol.*, 2002, 33(5), 478-83.

[6] Agaimy, A; Wunsch, PH; Hofstaedler, F; et al. Minute gastric Sclerosing stromal tumours (GIST tumourlets) are common in adults and frequently show c-KIT mutations. *Am J Surg Pathol*, 2007, 31,113.

[7] Miettinen, M; Sarlomo-Rikala, M; Lasota, J. Gastrointestinal stromal tumors: recent advances in understanding their biology. *Human Pathology*, 1999, 30,1213-1220.

[8] Barros, A; Linhares, E; Valadao, M; et al. Extragastrointestinal stromal tumours (EGIST): a series of case reports. *Hepatogastroenterology*, 2011, 58,865-868.

[9] Burkill, GJ; Badran, M; Al-Muderis, O; et al. Malignant gastrointestinal stromal tumor: distribution, imaging features, and pattern of metastatic spread. *Radiology*, 2003, 226, 527-532.

[10] Prakash, S; Sarran, L; Socci, N; et al. GIST in children and young adults: a clinicopathologic, molecular, and genomic study of 15 cases and review of literature. *J Pediatr Hematol Oncol*, 2005, 27,179-187.

[11] Miettinen, M; Lasota, J; Sobin, LH. Gastrointestinal stromal tumour of stomach in children and young adults: a clinicopathologic, immunohistochemical and genetic study of 44 cases with long term follow-up and review of literature. *Am J Surg Pathol*, 2005, 29,1973-81.

[12] Suster, S. Gastrointestinal stromal tumors. *Semin Diagn Pathol*, 1996, 13, 297-313.

[13] Miettinen, M; Sarlomo-Rikala, M; Sobin, LH; Lasota, J. Esophageal stromal tumor: a clinicopathologic, immunohistochemical and molecular genetic study of 17 cases and comparison with oesophageal leiomyoma and leiomyosarcoma. *Am J Surg Pathol*, 2000, 24, 211-22.

[14] Tio, TL; Tytgat, GN; den Hartog Jager, FC. Endoscopic ultrasonography for the evaluation of smooth muscle tumors in the upper gastrointestinal tract; an experience with 42 cases. *Gastrointestinal Endosc*, 1990, 36, 342.

[15] Ghanem, N; Altehoefer, C; Furtwängler, A; et al. Computed tomography in gastrointestinal stromal tumours. *Eur Radiol*, 2003, 13,1669.

[16] Chaudhry, UL; DeMatteo, RP. Advances in the surgical management of gastrointestinal stromal tumors. *Adv Surg*, 2011, 45, 197-209.

[17] Yu, MH; Lee, JM; Baek, JH; Han, JK; Choi, B. MRI features of gastrointestinal stromal tumors. *AJR Am J Roentgenol*, 2014, 203, 980-991.

[18] Kamiyama, Y; Aihara, R; Nakabayashi, T; et al. 18F-flurodeoxyglucose positron emission tomography: useful technique for predicting malignant potential of gastrointestinal stromal tumors. *World J Surg*, 2005, 29, 1429.

[19] Van den Abbeele, AD. The lessons of GIST-PET and PET/CT: a new paradigm for imaging. *Oncologist*, 2008, 13 suppl 2, 8-13.

[20] Fang, SH; Dong, DJ; Zhang, SZ; Jin, M. Angiographic findings of gastrointestinal stromal tumour. *World J Gastroenterol*, 2004, 10, 2905-7.

[21] Burhill, GJ; Barden, M; Al-Muderis, O; et al. Malignant gastrointestinal stromal tumor: Distribution, imaging features, and pattern of metastatic spread. *Radiology*, 2003, 226, 527-532.

[22] Sandrasegaran, K; Rajesh, A; Rushing, DA; Rydberg, J; Akisik, FM; Henley, JD. Gastrointestinal stromal tumors: CT and MRI findings. *Eur Radiol.*, 2005, 15(7), 1407-14.

[23] Levy, AD; Remotti, HE; Thompson, WM; Sobin, LH; Miettinen, M. Gastrointestinal stromal tumor: radiologic features with pathological correlation. *Radiographics*, 2003, 23, 283-304.

[24] Gu, M; Ghafari, S; Nguyen, PT; Lin, F. Cytologic diagnosis of gastrointestinal stromal tumors of the stomach by endoscopic ultrasound-guided fine-needle aspiration biopsy: cytomorphologic and immunohistochemical study of 12 cases. *Diagn Cytopathol*, 2001, 25, 343-350.

[25] Winant, AJ; Gollub, MJ; Shia, J; Antonescu, C; Bains, MS; Levine, MS. Imaging and clinicopathologic features of oesophageal gastrointestinal stromal tumors. *AJR Am J Roentgenol*, 2014, 203, 306-14.

[26] Nauert, TC; Zornoza, J; Ordonez, N. Gastric leiomyosarcoma. *AJR Am J Roentgenol*, 1982, 139, 291-297.

[27] Scatarige, JC; Fishman, EK; Jones, B; Cameron, JL; Sanders, RC; Siegelman, SS. Gastric leiomyosarcoma: CT observations. *J Comput Assist Tomogr*, 1985, 9, 320-327.

[28] Sharp, RM; Ansel, HJ; Keel, SB. Best cases from the AFIP: gastrointestinal stromal tumour. Armed Forces Institute of Pathology. *Radiographics*, 2001, 21, 1557-1560.

[29] Lee, SH; Ha, HK; Byun, JY; et al. Radiological features of leiomyomatous tumors of the colon and rectum. *J Comput Assist Tomagr*, 2000, 24, 407-412.

[30] Hama, Y; Okizuka, H; Odajima, K; Hayakawa, M; Kusano, S. Gastrointestinal stromal tumor of the rectum. *Eur Radiol*, 2001, 11, 216-219.

[31] Van den Berg, JC; van Heesewijk, JP; van Es, HW. Malignant stromal tumour of the rectum: findings at endorectal ultrasound and MRI. *Br J Radiol*, 2000, 73, 1010-1012.

[32] Zhu, J; Yang, Z; Tang, G; Wang, Z. Extragastrointestinal__stromal tumors: Computed tomography and magnetic resonance imaging findings. *Oncol Lett.*, 2015, 9(1), 201-208.

[33] Miettinen, M; Monihan, JM; Sarlomo–Rikala, M; et al. Gastrointestinal stromal tumors/smooth muscle tumors (GISTs) primary in the omentum and mesentery: clinicopathologic and immunohistochemical study of 26 cases. *Am J Surg Pathol*, 1999, 23,1109-1118.

[34] Minassian, SS; Frangipane, W; Polin, JI; Ellis, M. Leiomyomatosis peritonealis disseminata: a case report and literature review. *J Reprod Med*, 1986, 31, 997-1000.

[35] Ghrist, TD. Gastrointestinal involvement in neurofibromatosis. *Arch Internal Med*, 1963, 112, 357-362.

[36] Fuller, CE; Williams, GT. Gastrointestinal manifestations of type 1 neurofibromatosis (Von Recklinghausen's disease). *Histopathol*, 1991, 19, 1-11.

[37] Carney, JA. A triad of gastric epitheloid leiomyosarcoma, pulmonary chondroma and functioning extra adrenal paraganglioma: A five-year review. *Medicine (Baltimore)*, 1983, 62, 159-169.

[38] Heinrich, MC; Rubin, BP; Langley, BJ; et al. Biologic and genetic aspect of gastrointestinal stromal tumor: KIT activation and cytogenetic alteration. *Hum pathol*, 2002, 33, 484-495.
[39] Pfeffel, F; Stiglbauer, W; Depisch, D; Oberhuber, G; Raderer, M; Scheithauer, W. Coincidence of Crohn's disease and high risk gastrointestinal stromal tumor of the terminal ileum. *Digestion*, 1999, 60, 363-366.
[40] Changho, SC; Niece, JA; Saunders, C; Rivard, DC; Ahmed, A. Pediatric gastrointestinal stromal tumour in association with neuroblastoma. *APMIS*, 2011, 119, 164-6.
[41] Buckley, JA; Fishman, EK. CT evaluation of small bowel neoplasms: spectrum of disease. *Radiographics*, 1998, 18(2), 379-92.
[42] Sandrasegaran, K; Rajesh, A; Rydberg, J; Rushing, DA; Akisik, FM; Henley, JD. Gastrointestinal stromal tumors: clinical, radiologic, and pathologic features. *AJR Am J Roentgenol.*, 2005, 184(3), 803-11.
[43] Patnaik, S; Jyotsnarani, Y; Rammurti, S. Radiological features of metastatic gastrointestinal tumours. *J Clin Imaging Sci*, 2012, 2, 43.
[44] Chen, MY; Bechtold, RE; Savage, PD. Cystic changes in hepatic metastases from gastrointestinal stromal tumors (GISTs) treated with Gleevec (Imatinib mesylate). *AJR Am J Roentgenol*, 2002, 179, 1059-1062.
[45] Smiti, S; Rajagopal, K. CT mimics of peritoneal carcinomatosis. *Ind J Radiol Imag*, 2010, 20, 58-62.
[46] Kroep, JR; Bovee, JV; Van der Molen, AJ; Hogendoom, PC; Gelderblom, H. Extra-abdominal subcutaneous metastasis of a gastrointestinal stromal tumour: report of a case and review of the literature. *J Cutan Pathol*, 2009, 36, 565-9.
[47] Miettinen, M; Lasota, J. Gastrointestinal stromal tumors: review on morphology, molecular pathology, prognosis, differential diagnosis. *Arch Path Lab Med*, 2006, 130, 1466-1478.
[48] Pappo, AS; Janeway, K; Laquaglia, M; Kim, SY. Special considerations in_pediatric_gastrointestinal tumors. *J Surg Oncol.*, 2011, 104(8), 928-32.
[49] Janeway, KA; Kim, SY; Lodish, M; et al. Defects in succinate dehydrogenase in gastrointestinal stromal tumors lacking KIT and PDGFRA mutations. *Proc Natl Acad Sci USA*, 2011, 108, 314-318.
[50] Pappo, AS; Janeway, KA. Pediatric gastrointestinal stromal tumours. *Hematol Oncol Clin North Am*, 2009, 23,15-34.

[51] Dromain, C; De Baere, T; Elias, T; et al. Hepatic tumours treated with percutaneous radio-frequency ablation: CT and MRI imaging follow-up. Radiology 2002, 223,255-262.

In: Gastrointestinal Stromal Tumors in Adults ... ISBN: 978-1-63483-679-1
Editor: Atif A. Ahmed

Chapter 4

SURGICAL MANAGEMENT OF GASTROINTESTINAL STROMAL TUMORS

Rebecca A. Marmor and Jason K. Sicklick*
Division of Surgical Oncology and Department of Surgery,
Moores UCSD Cancer Center, University of California, San Diego,
UC San Diego Health System, CA, US

ABSTRACT

Surgical resection remains the principle treatment for Gastrointestinal Stromal Tumors (GIST). Several factors, including tumor number (i.e., localized, metastatic or multifocal disease), size, location, involvement of adjacent organs, proximity to critical structures, and presenting symptoms/signs are important to consider in operative decision-making. Whether an open, laparoscopic, or laparo-endoscopic approach is employed, the primary goal of surgical resection is to achieve total gross resection of disease with microscopically negative margins while maintaining an intact pseudocapsule, sparing adjacent organs uninvolved with tumor, and only resecting clinically positive lymph nodes. Furthermore, the patient's overall health status, coupled with symptoms should also be considered in these decisions. Finally, the use of neoadjvuant and adjuvant tyrosine kinase inhibitor therapies should be contemplated in

* Corresponding Author. Division of Surgical Oncology, Moores UCSD Cancer Center, University of California, San Diego, UC San Diego Health System, 3855 Health Sciences Drive, Mail Code 0987, La Jolla, CA 92093-0987; Tel: 858-822-6173, Fax: 858-228-5153, e-mail: jsicklick@ucsd.edu.

appropriately selected patients that may benefit in terms of a more limited resection, increasing the likelihood of resecting all gross disease, or decreasing the risk of recurrence. Given the multiple factors to consider in treatment decisions, a multidisciplinary approach is warranted in the care of all GIST patients.

INTRODUCTION

Gastrointestinal stromal tumors (GIST) originate from the interstitial cells of Cajal within the muscularis propria of the bowel. As a result, they can occur anywhere in the gastrointestinal tract. The most common tumor sites are the stomach (55.3%), small intestine (28.7%), colon (2.9%), rectum (2.1%), and esophagus (0.5%) [1]. GIST will either develop as endophytic or exophytic tumors within these locations. Based upon an analysis of 6,112 patients in the United States Surveillance, Epidemiology, and End-Results (SEER) database, tumors can range in size from small (e.g., ≤2-cm; 7.0%) to large (>10-cm; 24.2%). The remaining 52.3% range between 2- and 10-cm [1]. Over half of patients present with localized tumors, while nearly 15% present with regional disease and 22% present with metastatic disease. In the current era of targeted kinase inhibitors (TKIs), including imatinib (Gleevec, Novartis Pharmaceuticals) and aggressive surgical interventions, the prognosis for GIST patients can be quite favorable as compared to prior eras with current 5-year overall survival rates of 77%, 64%, and 41%, in patients with localized, regional, and metastatic disease, respectively [1].

RESECTABILITY

Several factors, including tumor number (i.e., metastatic or multifocal disease), size, location, involvement of adjacent organs, proximity to critical structures, and presenting symptoms are important considerations in operative decision-making. The patient's overall health status should also be considered. Given the multiple factors to consider, a multidisciplinary approach is warranted [2]. The following sections will provide further insight into this decision-making process.

I. GIST < 2-cm

Population-based studies have identified that asymptomatic "micro" GIST (<2-cm) can be found in approximately 20-30% of the elderly [3, 4]. These tumors have a distinct behavior from so-called "clinically relevant tumors" in terms of clinical and pathological factors. These "micro" GIST tend to have a lower proliferation rate, and are often characterized as hypocellular lesions composed of spindle cells, which demonstrate marked sclerosis [3]. For these tumors, abdominal/pelvic computed tomography (CT) and/or magnetic resonance imaging (MRI) should be performed to determine tumor location and the possible presence of metastatic disease [2, 5]. A biopsy should be obtained by endoscopic ultrasound with fine needle aspiration (EUS-FNA) or core needle biopsy to confirm the diagnosis and identify potential high-risk features including irregular border, cystic spaces, ulceration, echogenic foci, heterogeneity, and mitotic index $\geq$ 5/50 high power fields (HPF). Patients without high-risk features may be followed by periodic endoscopic surveillance for signs of transformation or until they become symptomatic [6]. The one exception to the aforementioned is that all rectovaginal GIST warrant resection, regardless of size, due to their increased risk of morbidity [5].

II. GIST>2-cm

A. Localized

For clearly resectable GIST>2-cm in a favorable anatomic location, abdominal/pelvic CT and/or MRI is recommended to identify potential metastases and help in operative planning. Resection is the preferred primary treatment for localized GIST>2-cm, as it remains the only chance for a cure [7]. Complete gross resection is possible in approximately 85% of patients with primary, localized disease without adjacent organ or vascular involvement that are situated in a favorable location (i.e., not the esophagus, duodenum, or rectum) [8]. In these cases, if patients are deemed to be acceptable operative candidates, neoadjuvant imatinib therapy is generally not recommended. On the other hand, if down-sizing the tumor will increase the ease of resection or limit the degree of resection (e.g., partial duodenal resection versus pancreaticoduodenectomy), then neoadjuvant imatinib should be considered.

Goals of Surgical Therapy

Margin Status

The primary goal of surgical resection is to achieve total gross resection of the tumor ideally with microscopically negative margins (i.e., R0) while maintaining an intact pseudocapsule [9]. Historically, the optimal margin of resection was an area of contention. A study by Gouiveia et al. [10] evaluated the influence of surgical margin status on outcomes. In this retrospective review of 113 patients with sporadic GIST, the percentage of recurrence was significantly lower in R0 resections (9%) than in R1 (microscopically positive margins, 27.8%) resections [10]. However, a large multi-institutional cohort study, which included 819 patients by McCarter *et al.* found no statistically significant difference in recurrence-free survival (RFS) at a median follow-up of 4 years between patients who had undergone R0 versus R1 resections [11]. In addition, among patients treated with placebo or adjuvant imatinib for 1 year, the overall risk of recurrence following an R1 resection was 39% and 35%, respectively, while it was only 27% among R0 resection patients in both groups. In subset analyses, the 3-year RFS rate for the R1 patients (N = 21) with tumor rupture was 60% versus 80% in the R1 patients without rupture (N = 51, HR 3.58, 95% CI: 1.65, 7.79, P = 0.001). Based on these findings, McCarter and colleagues concluded that the risk of recurrence is driven by the presence of tumor rupture or intra-peritoneal bleeding, but not microscopically positive margins. With these findings in mind, there is also no indication to re-operate after an R1 resection. On the other hand, grossly positive margin (R2) status clearly portends a worse prognosis with significantly shorter disease-specific survival rates [10]. Taken together, GIST must be handled carefully to decrease the risk of rupture, which is associated with an increased risk of recurrence, while attempting to achieve microscopically negative margins. With this in mind, an R1 resection may be tolerable for low-risk lesions with unfavorable tumor locations [12].

Organ Sparing Surgeries

While the matter of positive microscopic margins has been the subject of some debate, there is no clear evidence that negative microscopic margins result in improved survival [13, 14]. An analysis of 1,873 GIST cases in the SEER database showed similar outcomes for wedge and complete visceral resections [13]. However, resection of adjacent organs in order to obtain an R0 margin status led to increased morbidity [15]. As such, the current recommendation is to separate the tumor from adjacent organs if it is technically feasible and it does not compromise the tumor capsule or lead to tumor rupture in order to circumvent the morbidity associated with complex multi-visceral resections. As will be discussed later, situations such as this lend themselves to considering neoadjuvant imatinib therapy in order to downsize the tumor and allow for a higher chance of an R0 resection while sparing adjacent organs.

Role for Lymphadenectomy

Similar to most other sarcomas, lymphatic spread of GIST is quite rare and most commonly seen in younger patients. One review of 699 patients with GIST found a 1% rate of nodal involvement [16]. This most often occurred in patients under 40 years of age with epithelioid or mixed (e.g., epithelioid-spindle) histopathologies. A smaller case series by Naguib *et al.* found that among five patients with gastric GIST who underwent systematic lymphadenectomy for suspected lymph node involvement, none had microscopically positive nodes [17]. Finally, in a larger series with 200 patients, only 6% were found to have lymph node metastases [14]. As a result, lymphadenectomy is not routinely indicated in the surgical management of GIST [14, 18]. However, in cases where clinically or radiologically positive lymph node involvement is suspected, selective lymphadenectomy should be utilized

Location Dictates Operation

As GIST can develop anywhere along the gastrointestinal tract, a wide variety of surgical procedures may be employed in their resection. For example, a rectal GIST may necessitate a low anterior resection versus abdominoperineal resection for lower tumors and a duodenal GIST may warrant a partial duodenal resection versus pancreaticoduodenectomy. On the other hand, a small gastric GIST may require a simple wedge resection, while a larger gastric, or one located near the gastroesophageal junction may necessitate a more formal resection and reconstruction. Accordingly, an assortment of techniques is currently utilized in the resection of GIST.

Traditional surgical approaches to GIST include standard laparotomy and tumor resection based upon location. In a series of 140 gastric GIST reported by Fujimoto et al., only 3.5% of patients required total gastrectomy. The vast majority of patients underwent wedge resection (67.8%) or partial gastrectomy (27.9%) [19, 20]. In most surgical series, equivalent long-term results were obtained using a wedge resection or partial gastrectomy [19, 21-23].

In recent years, laparoscopic and combined laparoscopic-endoscopic surgical approaches have gained popularity because quite often only a wedge resection without reconstruction is required. Therefore, laparoscopic techniques are now well-established for the resection of gastric GIST ranging in size from 3.4- to 10-cm without additional risk of complications or recurrence [24-26]. Furthermore, this approach has been associated with shorter hospital stays, less pain, improved cosmesis, and decreased morbidity [24, 27]. These benefits are in the absence of increased rates of local/port site recurrences [24], or effects upon survival [28]. A laparoscopic approach can also be utilized for tumors located in the jejunum or ileum [21]. Tumors larger than 5 cm may be resected using a laparoscopic assisted technique with a hand port. Similar approaches may be utilized for colonic tumors. In contrast to the minimally invasive approaches with limited resections that have been previously discussed, tumors near the gastroesophageal junction have historically warranted proximal or total gastrectomies [21]. However, recent case series have demonstrated the utility of combined laparoscopic and endoscopic approaches, especially for endophytic tumors adjacent to the gastroesophageal junction, along the lesser curve of the stomach, or arising from the posterior wall of the stomach [29-31]. The laparo-endoscopic technique offers several advantages to the surgeon including: 1) an extra working port in the endoscope to minimize instrument changes, 2) a hand-activated, auto-cleaning capability for the camera lens, 3) improved ability to visualize remote locations in the abdomen given the endoscope's flexibility [31]. Similar combined approaches have been utilized for rectal GIST [32]. The smaller rectal GIST may be removed by full-thickness transanal or trans-sphincteric resections if they are located in the lower one-third of the rectum [33]. However, care must be taken when utilizing this approach, as it has been associated with higher microscopically positive margins and higher recurrence rates [34, 35]. Finally, a word of caution is necessary when consider any laparoscopic approach for resecting GIST. If the tumor appears to be cystic or very necrotic on imaging, there may be a higher risk of rupture with such an approach. In these scenarios, an open approach may be more prudent. Taken together, personalized surgical approach must be tailored to each patient based upon several factors including tumor related factors, the surgeon's technical skill set, and patient-related factors.

B. Locally Advanced

Tumors which are initially deemed unresectable have the potential to become resectable after neoadjuvant imatinib therapy [36]. While GIST rarely invade adjacent structures, this is not always the case. When adherence to adjacent organs is identified, an *en bloc* resection is favored to prevent intra-abdominal dissemination of tumor, which is associated with high recurrence rates [37, 38]. Current evidence suggests that patients with locally advanced tumors at initial diagnosis are best treated with neoadjuvant imatinib, which may allow for tumor downsizing and the completion of a less morbid, or possibly even less invasive, operation [39]. Several studies support its use in patients with borderline resectable primary GIST. Tielen et al. evaluated 57 patients with locally advanced primary GIST who received neoadjuvant imatinib for a median of 8 months. Imatinib caused tumor reduction (median 49%) and enabled rupture-free R0 resection in 84% of patients. The 5-year progression-free survival (PFS) and overall survival (OS) were 77% and 88%, respectively [40]. Additionally in patients with advanced primary GIST who received neoadjuvant imatinib for up to 12 months, 11 of 14 (79%) subsequently underwent complete resection with favorable prognoses [i.e., 4-year OS of 100% and 4- year disease-free survival (DFS) of 64%] [41]. Neoadjuvant imatinib can also facilitate resection of regionally advanced, borderline resectable GIST [42]. Although rare, omental and mesenteric GIST also warrant complete en bloc resection, including involved adjacent organs [43]. Taken together, neoadjuvant imatinib can be helpful in treating borderline or initially unresectable tumors, in addition to consideration in patients with poorly situated GIST (e.g., esophageal, duodenal or rectal) as previously discussed.

Before, during, and after a course of neoadjuvant imatinib, positron emission tomography (*PET*)-CT scanning can be utilized in order to assess response to treatment based upon standard uptake values (SUV) and CT imaging characteristics. These are favored over traditional CT alone because they detect changes earlier [44]. Usually, the maximum tumor response occurs within 6-12 months of treatment, without further benefit from continuing treatment. Therefore, according to National Comprehensive Cancer Network (NCCN) and European Society Medical Oncology (ESMO) guidelines, the treatment duration should be based upon the individual patient's tumor response. When stable disease has been achieved, an operation should be performed [45]. In summary, for large, locally advanced GIST in which resection carries significant risk of morbidity or functional deficit, and in those patients with poorly positioned tumors that are marginally resectable or unresectable neoadjuvant therapy should be administered in a multi-disciplinary fashion [2].

C. Metastatic Disease

Approximately 50% of patients who undergo GIST resection will develop recurrent disease [14], at which time approximately two-thirds will have liver metastases and half will have peritoneal disease [46]. The role of neoadjuvant imatinib and/or cytoreductive surgery for metastatic and/or recurrent GIST is still being elucidated. Several trials comparing TKIs to cytoreductive surgery have failed to adequately accrue patients. However, there is reasonably strong rationale for the use of TKIs in combination with surgical resection in the management of metastatic disease. A study by Tielen et al. examining 55 patients with metastatic GIST underwent surgery after a median 16 months of TKI therapy (range, 3-72 months) [47]. Postoperatively, the rate of tumor recurrence or progression was lower in patients who responded to preoperative TKI therapy (48%) than in those who did not (85%). Although nearly all patients who undergo excision of metastases ultimately experience recurrence [46], initial response to combined preoperative TKI therapy and complete resection correlate with improved PFS and OS [47]. A recent series by Bischof *et al.* examining the outcomes of patients with advanced GIST, found that 3-year RFS and OS rates among patients with recurrent/metastatic GIST were 49% and 82%, respectively. The study also found that lack of adjuvant TKI was associated with worse outcomes [48].

The first prospective large trial of neoadjuvant imatinib sponsored by the RTOG evaluated the effectiveness and toxicity of preoperative imatinib, administered for 8-12 weeks, followed by surgical resection to debulk all tumor [49]. This was followed by 2 years of adjuvant imatinib. They found that R0 and R1 resection had no substantial impact on tumor progression, when compared with patients who had no resection. Despite this finding, the clear benefits of debulking included the obviation/delay of drug resistance and the prevention of complications from a large metastatic burden.

While surgical cytoreduction can also be used to enhance disease control and remove residual disease, subjecting patients to extensive abdominal surgery in the setting of chemo-responsive or limited, stable metastatic disease in the absence of symptoms may not necessarily always be indicated. Therefore, combined with neoadjuvant imatinib therapy, metastatectomy can be effective in selected patients. In a retrospective study, seven patients with advanced/recurrent GIST underwent radical resection of liver (N = 4), peritoneal (N = 1), liver and peritoneal (N = 1), or liver and lymph node (N = 1) metastases upon best response to preoperative imatinib; imatinib was then continued for a median of 26 months. The 2-year PFS was 64.4% [50]. As a result, in patients with metastatic disease, current recommendations include assessment by a multidisciplinary team with medical and surgical oncology expertise [2].

D. Symptomatic GIST

Symptomatic GIST is an indication for urgent/emergent resection. A case series examining 94 patients who presented with emergent symptomatic tumors found the most common symptoms included: upper gastrointestinal bleeding (49%), intestinal obstruction (28%), and intraperitoneal bleeding (15%) [51]. Of the 94 patients who presented acutely, 90 underwent immediate resection. Eight-six (95.6%) patients received complete macroscopic resection, while 11 patients went on to develop metastases or recurrent disease. The 5-year OS rate for all patients was 81.4% and the 5-year DFS rate was 64.5%. A similar, but smaller series, studying acute presentations of GIST in the elderly found that among 12 elderly patients, 41.7% presented with gastrointestinal bleeding and 16.6% presented with perforation [52]. All 12 patients underwent emergency operations. At a mean follow-up of 21 months, 11 patients (91.6%) were alive and disease-free. Based upon the studies, early surgical intervention is recommended in patients with some symptomatic tumors who present with bleeding, obstruction, or intractable pain. In cases where extensive disease exists, but the patient presents with one of the three aforementioned presentations, an incomplete cytoreduction should only be carried out as a palliative therapy [14].

Conclusion

Having been largely resistant to chemotherapeutics, historically, surgical resection evolved as the mainstay of treatment for GIST. While surgery remains critical for a chance at cure, the advent of tyrosine kinase inhibitors, in combination with increasingly sensitive imaging technologies as well as a growing number of minimally invasive surgical approaches have contributed to the evolution of treatment options and algorithms for the management of patients with GIST.

REFERENCES

[1] Ma GL, Murphy JD, Martinez ME, Sicklick JK. Epidemiology of Gastrointestinal Stromal Tumors in the Era of Histology Codes: Results of a Population-Based Study. *Cancer Epidemiol Biomarkers Prev* 2015;24(1):298-302.

[2] Group EESNW. Gastrointestinal stromal tumors: ESMO Clinical Practice Guidelines for diagnosis, treatment and follow-up. *Ann Oncol* 2012; 23 Suppl 7: vii49-55.

[3] Agaimy A, Wunsch PH, Hofstaedter F et al. Minute gastric sclerosing stromal tumors (GIST tumorlets) are common in adults and frequently show c-KIT mutations. *Am J Surg Pathol* 2007; 31: 113-120.

[4] Kawanowa K, Sakuma Y, Sakurai S et al. High incidence of microscopic gastrointestinal stromal tumors in the stomach. *Hum Pathol* 2006; 37: 1527-1535.

[5] Casali PG, Blay JY, ESMO/CONTICANET/EUROBONET Consensus Panel of Experts. Gastrointestinal stromal tumours: ESMO Clinical Practice Guidelines for diagnosis, treatment and follow-up. *Ann Oncol* 2010; 21 Suppl 5: v98-102.

[6] Sicklick JK, Lopez NE. Optimizing surgical and imatinib therapy for the treatment of gastrointestinal stromal tumors. *J Gastrointest Surg* 2013; 17: 1997-2006.

[7] DeMatteo RP. The GIST of targeted cancer therapy: a tumor (gastrointestinal stromal tumor), a mutated gene (c-kit), and a molecular inhibitor (STI571). *Ann Surg Oncol* 2002; 9: 831-839.

[8] Chaudhry UI, DeMatteo RP. Management of resectable gastrointestinal stromal tumor. *Hematol Oncol Clin North Am* 2009; 23: 79-96, viii.

[9] Ng EH, Pollock RE, Munsell MF et al. Prognostic factors influencing survival in gastrointestinal leiomyosarcomas. Implications for surgical management and staging. *Ann Surg* 1992; 215: 68-77.

[10] Gouveia AM, Pimenta AP, Capelinha AF et al. Surgical margin status and prognosis of gastrointestinal stromal tumor. *World J Surg* 2008; 32: 2375-2382.

[11] McCarter MD, Antonescu CR, Ballman KV et al. Microscopically positive margins for primary gastrointestinal stromal tumors: analysis of risk factors and tumor recurrence. *J Am Coll Surg* 2012; 215: 53-59; discussion 59-60.

[12] Eisenberg BL, Harris J, Blanke CD et al. Phase II trial of neoadjuvant/adjuvant imatinib mesylate (IM) for advanced primary and

metastatic/recurrent operable gastrointestinal stromal tumor (GIST): early results of RTOG 0132/ACRIN 6665. *J Surg Oncol* 2009; 99: 42-47.
[13] Perez EA, Gutierrez JC, Jin X et al. Surgical outcomes of gastrointestinal sarcoma including gastrointestinal stromal tumors: a population-based examination. *J Gastrointest Surg* 2007; 11: 114-125.
[14] DeMatteo RP, Lewis JJ, Leung D et al. Two hundred gastrointestinal stromal tumors: recurrence patterns and prognostic factors for survival. *Ann Surg* 2000; 231: 51-58.
[15] Martin RC, 2nd, Jaques DP, Brennan MF, Karpeh M. Achieving RO resection for locally advanced gastric cancer: is it worth the risk of multiorgan resection? *J Am Coll Surg* 2002; 194: 568-577.
[16] Agaimy A, Wunsch PH. Lymph node metastasis in gastrointestinal stromal tumours (GIST) occurs preferentially in young patients < or = 40 years: an overview based on our case material and the literature. *Langenbecks Arch Surg* 2009; 394: 375-381.
[17] Naguib SF, Zaghloul AS, El Marakby H. Gastrointestinal stromal tumors (GIST) of the stomach: retrospective experience with surgical resection at the National Cancer Institute. *J Egypt Natl Canc Inst* 2008; 20: 80-89.
[18] Shiu MH, Farr GH, Papachristou DN, Hajdu SI. Myosarcomas of the stomach: natural history, prognostic factors and management. *Cancer* 1982; 49: 177-187.
[19] Fujimoto Y, Nakanishi Y, Yoshimura K, Shimoda T. Clinicopathologic study of primary malignant gastrointestinal stromal tumor of the stomach, with special reference to prognostic factors: analysis of results in 140 surgically resected patients. *Gastric Cancer* 2003; 6: 39-48.
[20] Miettinen M, Sobin LH, Lasota J. Gastrointestinal stromal tumors of the stomach: a clinicopathologic, immunohistochemical, and molecular genetic study of 1765 cases with long-term follow-up. *Am J Surg Pathol* 2005; 29: 52-68.
[21] Heinrich MC, Corless CL. Gastric GI stromal tumors (GISTs): the role of surgery in the era of targeted therapy. *J Surg Oncol* 2005; 90: 195-207; discussion 207.
[22] Aparicio T, Boige V, Sabourin JC et al. Prognostic factors after surgery of primary resectable gastrointestinal stromal tumours. *Eur J Surg Oncol* 2004; 30: 1098-1103.

[23] Mochizuki Y, Kodera Y, Ito S et al. Treatment and risk factors for recurrence after curative resection of gastrointestinal stromal tumors of the stomach. *World J Surg* 2004; 28: 870-875.

[24] Novitsky YW, Kercher KW, Sing RF, Heniford BT. Long-term outcomes of laparoscopic resection of gastric gastrointestinal stromal tumors. *Ann Surg* 2006; 243: 738-745; discussion 745-737.

[25] Sexton JA, Pierce RA, Halpin VJ et al. Laparoscopic gastric resection for gastrointestinal stromal tumors. *Surg Endosc* 2008; 22: 2583-2587.

[26] Sokolich J, Galanopoulos C, Dunn E et al. Expanding the indications for laparoscopic gastric resection for gastrointestinal stromal tumors. *JSLS* 2009; 13: 165-169.

[27] Otani Y, Ohgami M, Igarashi N et al. Laparoscopic wedge resection of gastric submucosal tumors. *Surg Laparosc Endosc Percutan Tech* 2000; 10: 19-23.

[28] Karakousis GC, Singer S, Zheng J et al. Laparoscopic versus open gastric resections for primary gastrointestinal stromal tumors (GISTs): a size-matched comparison. *Ann Surg Oncol* 2011; 18: 1599-1605.

[29] Henckens T, Van de Putte D, Van Renterghem K et al. Laparoendoscopic single-site gastrectomy for a gastric GIST using double-bended instruments. *J Laparoendosc Adv Surg Tech* A 2010; 20: 469-471.

[30] Hirano Y, Watanabe T, Uchida T et al. Laparoendoscopic single site partial resection of the stomach for gastrointestinal stromal tumor. *Surg Laparosc Endosc Percutan Tech* 2010; 20: 262-264.

[31] Barajas-Gamboa JS, Acosta G, Savides TJ et al. Laparo-endoscopic transgastric resection of gastric submucosal tumors. *Surg Endosc* 2015 Aug;29(8):2149-57..

[32] Maker AV. A technique for laparoendoscopic resection of posterior fundic gastric GISTs without need for a gastrotomy. *Ann Surg Oncol* 2013; 20: 4238.

[33] Hellan M, Maker VK. Transvaginal excision of a large rectal stromal tumor: an alternative. *Am J Surg* 2006; 191: 121-123.

[34] Dong C, Jun-Hui C, Xiao-Jun Y et al. Gastrointestinal stromal tumors of the rectum: Clinical, pathologic, immunohistochemical characteristics and prognostic analysis. *Scand J Gastroenterol* 2007; 42: 1221-1229.

[35] Changchien CR, Wu MC, Tasi WS et al. Evaluation of prognosis for malignant rectal gastrointestinal stromal tumor by clinical parameters and immunohistochemical staining. *Dis Colon Rectum* 2004; 47: 1922-1929.

[36] Fanta PT, Sicklick JK, Betz BL, Peterson MR. In Vivo Imatinib Sensitivity in a Patient With GI Stromal Tumor Bearing a PDGFRA Deletion DIM842-844. *J Clin Oncol* 2015 Mar 10;33(8):e41-4..

[37] Joensuu H, Eriksson M, Hall KS et al. Risk factors for gastrointestinal stromal tumor recurrence in patients treated with adjuvant imatinib. *Cancer* 2014 Aug 1;120(15):2325-33.

[38] Rutkowski P, Bylina E, Wozniak A et al. Validation of the Joensuu risk criteria for primary resectable gastrointestinal stromal tumour - the impact of tumour rupture on patient outcomes. *Eur J Surg Oncol* 2011; 37: 890-896.

[39] An HJ, Ryu MH, Ryoo BY et al. The effects of surgical cytoreduction prior to imatinib therapy on the prognosis of patients with advanced GIST. *Ann Surg Oncol* 2013; 20: 4212-4218.

[40] Tielen R, Verhoef C, van Coevorden F et al. Surgical treatment of locally advanced, non-metastatic, gastrointestinal stromal tumours after treatment with imatinib. *Eur J Surg Oncol* 2013; 39: 150-155.

[41] Doyon C, Sideris L, Leblanc G et al. Prolonged Therapy with Imatinib Mesylate before Surgery for Advanced Gastrointestinal Stromal Tumor Results of a Phase II Trial. *Int J Surg Oncol* 2012; 2012: 761576.

[42] Koontz MZ, Visser BM, Kunz PL. Neoadjuvant imatinib for borderline resectable GIST. *J Natl Compr Canc Netw* 2012; 10: 1477-1482; quiz 1482.

[43] Blay JY, Bonvalot S, Casali P et al. Consensus meeting for the management of gastrointestinal stromal tumors. Report of the GIST Consensus Conference of 20-21 March 2004, under the auspices of ESMO. *Ann Oncol* 2005; 16: 566-578.

[44] Goldstein D, Tan BS, Rossleigh M et al. Gastrointestinal stromal tumours: correlation of F-FDG gamma camera-based coincidence positron emission tomography with CT for the assessment of treatment response--an AGITG study. *Oncology* 2005; 69: 326-332.

[45] Bumming P, Andersson J, Meis-Kindblom JM et al. Neoadjuvant, adjuvant and palliative treatment of gastrointestinal stromal tumours (GIST) with imatinib: a centre-based study of 17 patients. *Br J Cancer* 2003; 89: 460-464.

[46] Chaudhry UI, DeMatteo RP. Advances in the surgical management of gastrointestinal stromal tumor. *Adv Surg* 2011; 45: 197-209.

[47] Tielen R, Verhoef C, van Coevorden F et al. Surgery after treatment with imatinib and/or sunitinib in patients with metastasized

gastrointestinal stromal tumors: is it worthwhile? *World J Surg Oncol* 2012; 10: 111.

[48] Bischof DA, Kim Y, Blazer DG, 3rd et al. Surgical management of advanced gastrointestinal stromal tumors: an international multi-institutional analysis of 158 patients. *J Am Coll Surg* 2014; 219: 439-449.

[49] Wang D, Zhang Q, Blanke CD et al. Phase II trial of neoadjuvant/adjuvant imatinib mesylate for advanced primary and metastatic/recurrent operable gastrointestinal stromal tumors: long-term follow-up results of Radiation Therapy Oncology Group 0132. *Ann Surg Oncol* 2012; 19: 1074-1080.

[50] Nannini M, Pantaleo MA, Maleddu A et al. Duration of adjuvant treatment following radical resection of metastases from gastrointestinal stromal tumours. *Oncol Lett* 2012; 3: 677-681.

[51] Sorour MA, Kassem MI, Ghazal Ael H et al. Gastrointestinal stromal tumors (GIST) related emergencies. *Int J Surg* 2014; 12: 269-280.

[52] Marano L, Arru GM, Piras M et al. Surgical management of acutely presenting gastrointestinal stromal tumors of the stomach among elderly: experience of an emergency surgery department. *Int J Surg* 2014; 12 Suppl 1: S145-147.

In: Gastrointestinal Stromal Tumors in Adults ... ISBN: 978-1-63483-679-1
Editor: Atif A. Ahmed

Chapter 5

PATHOLOGIC DIAGNOSIS OF GASTROINTESTINAL STROMAL TUMORS

Atif A. Ahmed*
University of Missouri,
Department of Pathology and Laboratory Medicine,
Kansas City, MO, US

ABSTRACT

Gastrointestinal stromal tumors (GIST) are believed to arise through oncogenic mutations in the interstitial cells of Cajal, the pacemaker cells of the gastrointestinal tract. Such tumors are predominantly found in the stomach and small intestine although they may occur in part of the gut wall as well as extraintestinal sites. The pathologic diagnosis of GIST primarily depends on the examination of tissue specimens with histology and immunohistochemistry. Regardless of patient's age and location, GIST tumors are characterized by similar gross and microscopic details. The diagnosis is suspected by identifying the spindle cell, epithelioid or mixed stromal morphology and confirmed by immunohistochmical staining with CD117, CD34 and/or DOG1. Molecular diagnostic tests for Kit and PDGFR mutations are becoming increasingly available to confirm the diagnosis and aid in patient's management. Prognostic markers should be identified during routine pathologic examination and molecular testing.

* Email: aahmed@cmh.edu.

INTRODUCTION

Gastrointestinal stromal tumors (GIST) are the most common mesenchymal tumors in the GI tract [1]. Although they can occur anywhere in the gastrointestinal tract, including the omentum, mesentery, and retroperitoneum, they are most common in the stomach where they may affect any part of the stomach wall. It is now well established that GIST tumors are derived from the intestinal cells of Cajal (ICC) [1, 2]. These cells are normally found in the gut wall; specifically in the submucosa, the muscularis propria layers, and surrounding the ganglion cells of the myenteric plexus, and are recognized as the gut pacemaker cells that regulate intestinal motility. GIST tumors arise through oncogenic mutations that most commonly occur in the *KIT* gene resulting in activation and expression of the KIT protein in the majority of cases [3, 4].

PATHOGENESIS

The most frequent mutation in GIST is that of the KIT receptor tyrosine kinase. KIT is highly expressed in ICC and is responsible for their oncogenic transformation. Upon binding its ligand, stem cell factor, the KIT receptor dimerizes and initiates a signal transduction phosphorylation cascade that results in the regulation of cell growth [5]. ETV1, an ETS family transcription factor, is also highly expressed in a subtype of ICCs, being a major regulator of their development. Recent studies have revealed that ETV1 is required for GIST initiation and proliferation in vivo [6, 7]. Activated KIT cooperates with ETV1 to promote and maintain GIST tumorigenesis. Through a positive feedback circuit involving MAP kinase activation, KIT stabilizes the ETV1 protein and ETV1 positively regulates KIT expression. GIST arises from those ICCs with high levels of endogenous ETV1 expression that undergo activating KIT mutations. Activation of KIT results in activation of MAP kinase, which in turn, through the positive feedback, maintains and accentuates KIT and ETV1 expression [7, 8]. This oncogenic program, coupled by inactivation of tumor suppressor genes such as dystrophin [9], is presumed to be the main pathway of GIST tumorigenesis.

GIST with wild type KIT undergo mutations of other genes such as platelet-derived growth factor –alpha (*PDGFRA*), succinate dehydrogenase complex, *BRAF/RAS*, and *NF*1 genes [10]. These tumors arise from different unknown mechanisms that eventually lead to interaction and activation of the KIT protein. The insulin growth factor pathway and other pathway proteins may be activated in a subset of these tumors [11]. Still, approximately 5% of GIST do not harbor mutations in any of the known genes. Such cases have been named quadruple wild type GIST [12].

Diagnostic Specimens

Both endoscopic biopsies and bowel resection specimens can be delivered to the laboratory for histologic diagnosis. Small lesions (<2 cm) are difficult to biopsy and often require bowel resection for diagnosis [13]. A portion of the fresh specimen is usually stored away and frozen for molecular genetic studies. There are currently no specific guidelines addressing the use of intraoperative consultation services during surgery. Pathology specimens are commonly fixed in 10% formaldehyde; however there are no published studies or guidelines addressing the optimal duration of fixation. Bouin fixative should be avoided as it can impair molecular analysis from paraffin-embedded tissue. The final diagnostic pathology report should ideally describe the gross and microscopic appearance of the tumor and mention all possible prognostic parameters, such as tumor size, mitotic rate, or presence of invasion [13, 14].

Cytology specimens from ultrasound-guided fine needle aspiration or other techniques such as brushing or lavage can also be utilized in the diagnosis of GIST. Most of the studies commented on the utility of such approach in GIST of the stomach. Several authors have documented good outcome in large tumors and lesions less than 2 cm. While the accuracy of morphology and immunohistochemistry (IHC) is less 90% in most reported series, an increase in specimen yield and improved diagnostic accuracy are reported in GIST with gastric locations, large tumor size and presence of on-site cytopathology assessment tools [15].

Gross Appearance

GIST tumors may be single or multiple in a stomach or bowel resection and often are well-circumscribed without a true capsule [16]. In the pediatric population, they frequently are present as multiple nodules, and the tumor greatest dimension will then be difficult to measure (Figure 1A). The tumor may be exophytic subserosal, intramural or uncommonly polypoid submucosal mass associated with surface ulceration and bleeding. Small GIST are commonly subserosal or intramural. Tumors have soft or rubbery consistency and larger tumors may have cystic degeneration, hemorrhage or necrosis. It important to note the accurate localization of the tumor, as gastric location is associated with favorable prognosis. Gross features suggesting malignancy or high risk should be also noted such as large tumor size, mucosal ulceration, and invasion of adjacent organs [17].

Microscopic Appearance

Regardless of their location and age presentation, GIST share common histologic features with basic cell morphologies: spindled, epithelioid or mixed (Figure 1). The spindle cell morphology is the most common and cells may show paranuclear vacuolization, nuclear palisading and/or a plexiform growth pattern. Tumors in the small bowel may show brightly eosinophilic fibrillary structures known as "skenoid fibers". Epithelioid GIST morphology is seen in 20% of cases most often consist of round vacuolated or clear cells arranged in nests or sheets [18-22]. Areas with signet-cell appearance may also be present as well as vascular stroma with myxoid areas [23, 24]. Cellularity and stromal changes vary greatly giving rise to a variety of appearances that include sclerosing, dyscohesive, sarcomatous and hypercellular [14]. Pleomorphism is uncommon and usually associated with epithelioid morphology and malignant potential. However, mild pleomorphism may occasionally occur in benign tumors. Mitotic rate is variable and generally low. Areas of dedifferentiation associated with cellular anaplasia and loss of KIT immunoreactivity have recently been reported [25].

Needle Aspiration Specimens

Cytopathologic specimens of spindle GIST usually reveal spindle-shaped cells with scant, lightly eosinophilic cytoplasm, elongated/oval plump nuclei and mild pleomorphism. The chromatin is clumped with indistinct nucleoli [26, 27]. Alternatively, tight aggregates or loosely cohesive epithelioid cells can be found in epithelioid GIST. Suspicious morphology can be confirmed by cell blocks and immunocytochemistry [28, 29].

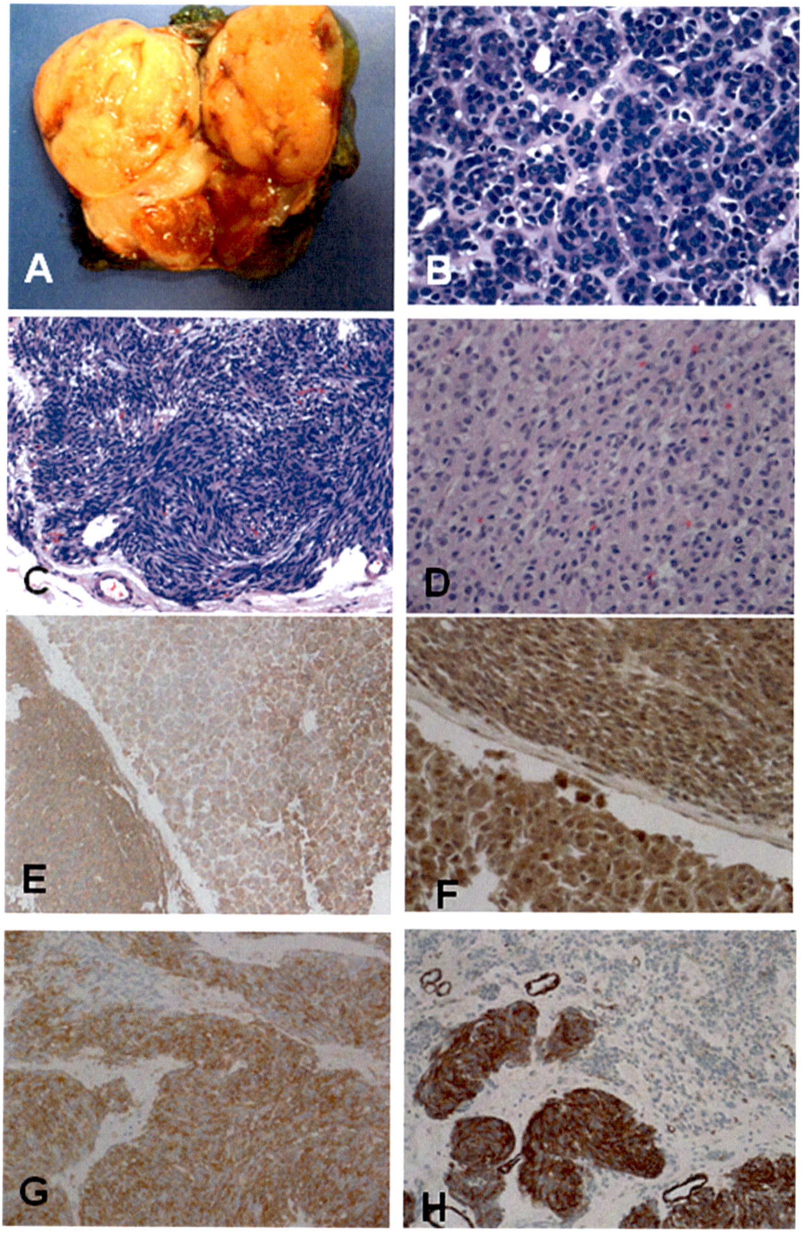

Figure 1.

A. Gross appearance of multi-nodular GIST with fleshy soft yellow appearance.

B. Epithelioid GIST infiltrating the muscularis propria (H&E x100).

C. Spindle GIST revealing nuclear palisading and whorl formation (H&E x100).

D. Spindle GIST tumor cells with paranuclear vacuolization (H&E x200).
E. Immunohistochemistry for CD117 reveals variation of staining intensity in spindle cell and epithelioid areas (x100).
F. Immunohistochemistry for PDGFRA revealing diffuse positive staining (x200).
G. CD34 immunohistochemistry is positive in the majority of cases (x200).
H. Staining for h-caldesmon may also be positive in focal areas (x200).

IMMUNOHISTOCHEMISTRY

The most consistent IHC markers utilized in the diagnosis of GIST and differentiating it from other entities are KIT (CD117) and DOG-1, which are found in the vast majority (>95%) of GISTs [18-22]. Immunohistochemical positivity for KIT (CD117) can be cytoplasmic, membranous or paranuclear dot-like pattern (Figure 1). The staining can sometimes be focal or weak, particularly in some epithelioid stomach tumors [5, 8]. KIT expression is present in most tumors regardless of the mutation status. In those rare situations where KIT is not expressed, immunohistochemistry for DOG1 is useful. More than 80% of cases also express CD34 which can also help establish the diagnosis. Other immunostaining markers are less frequent and include smooth muscle actin and h-caldesmon. Immunoreactivity for desmin, cytokeratins and S-100 is rare. Vimentin is non-specifically expressed as in all mesenchymal tumors [30].

THE DIFFERENTIAL DIAGNOSIS

The histologic appearance of GIST is not specific and can also be seen in other mesenchymal tumors of the gut such as desmoid fibromatosis, leiomyomas, leiomyosarcomas, gastrointestinal schwannomas, inflammatory myofibroblastic tumor, inflammatory fibroid polyps, and solitary fibrous tumors [31, 32]. Epithelioid GIST may also be confused with carcinoma. These tumors mimic GIST and can be a source of confusion especially in needle biopsy specimens and uncommon locations [33]. Depending on the specimen size, GIST can easily be differentiated from other entities with the use of imunohistochemical stains and molecular analysis. Knowledge of the tumor location also helps in narrowing this differential. Kaposi sarcoma is detected on mucosal biopsies, whereas inflammatory fibroid polyp is nearly always in the submucosa. On the other hand, (GISTs) are generally centered in the muscularis propria, similar to schwannomas. True leiomyomas are most common in the esophagus and colon where GIST is more common in the stomach and small intestine. Mesenteric lesions are usually found in the small bowel mesentery. Mesenschymal polyps can also be a differential diagnosis for GIST in the colon [34].

GIST can easily be differentiated from these tumors by using an IHC panel of that includes CD117. Most of the other mesenchymal tumors of the gut are negative for CD117 and CD34 or rarely exhibit very focal staining. The confusion arises in the differentiation of KIT-negative GIST from other tumors. Positivity for CD34 should not be relied upon, as GIST of the small bowel are less frequently positive [35]. In these situations, DOG1 immunohistochemistry will be of tremendous help. In this context, it is worth mentioning that monophasic synovial sarcoma and smooth muscle tumors may also rarely be positive for DOG1 and hence can be confused with GIST [36]. Alk immunohistochemistry can differentiate inflammatory myofibroblastic tumor from GIST.

Molecular Genetics

DNA specimens can be extracted from fresh, frozen or paraffin-embedded tissue. Detection of mutations of the *KIT* and *PDGFRA* genes is important in the diagnosis and assessing the prognosis of the patient [37, 38]. *KIT* mutations are more common in spindle cell tumors than epithelioid types while tumors with *PDGFRA* mutations frequently have epithelioid morphology and follow a benign course [39, 40]. Mutations of KIT or PDGFRA are not entirely specific for GIST and can occur in other tumors as well. Of the gut mesenchymal lesions, inflammatory fibroid polyp can also harbor n mutations in the *PDGFRA* gene [41, 42]. Mutations are more common in adults than children who harbor *KIT* or *PDGFRA* mutations in only 15% of patients [43]. GIST that are wild type for *KIT* and *PDGFRA* should be screened for *SDH* and *BRAF* mutations, where they have been described in a minority of cases [44-46]. Mutational analysis is commonly performed with polymerase chain reaction or DNA sequencing methods.

Recently, mutations in the tumor suppressor gene, succinate dehydrogenase (*SDH*), have been described in GIST of the stomach, and include mutations involving subunits A, B, C or D of the SDH complex. These mutations disrupt the expression of the corresponding mitochondrial enzyme predisposing to the development of tumors. SDH-deficient GIST occur in the pediatric population where most of the cases are also wild type for *KIT* and *PDGFRA*. This type of GIST constitutes a small subgroup of gastric GIST and often exhibits an indolent chronic course. SDH-deficient GIST have characteristic morphologic features including multinodular gastric wall involvement, multi-focality, common lymphovascular invasion, and occasional lymph node metastases [44, 45].

There is poor correlation between mutational analysis results and immunohistochemical studies of the mutated proteins. Expression of the KIT protein (CD117) also occurs in most of cases that are wild type for *KIT*. Immunohistochemistry for PDGFR-alpha may give positive results in GIST but has not been well-characterized and often yields non-specific diffuse staining. Similarly, immunostaining for BRAF reveals non-specific results that do not correlate with the mutational status of the gene. The opposite can be said about the correlation between immunohistochemistry and mutational analysis of the SDH complex. Loss of immunohistochemical staining for SDH subunit B correlates fairly with SDH-deficient status [45]. Recently, mutations in SDH subunit A have also been identified and correlates with the immunohistochemical loss of the SDHA protein.

Prognosis

The diagnostic pathology report should yield useful information regarding the tumor grade and patient's prognosis. Tumor size, mitotic index, anatomic location, tumor rupture and disease-free interval are the classic clinic-pathologic features used to predict the clinical course of patients who undergo complete gross resection [47, 48]. Tumors with size > 5cm and >5 mitotic cells per 50 high power field are more likely to metastasize [49, 50]. Tumors in the small intestine, even if associated with epithelioid morphology, tend to have a worse prognosis than those in the stomach. Vascular invasion and atypical mitotic figures are also good predictors of adverse malignant potential [21]. Factors associated with disease progression are combined to categorize patients as very low, low, intermediate and high risk. A recent study has revealed the clinicopathologic risk stratification carries a correlation with long term disease-free survival [51]. Recent studies have also addressed the significance of the mutational profile of tumor and its relation to the disease prognosis. Patients with *PDGFRA* mutations had more favorable RFS than those with *KIT* mutations. Similarly, patients whose tumors harbor mutations in exon 11 of the *KIT* gene tend to have better disease-free survival than patients with exon 9 mutations [50, 52].

The majority of pediatric GIST tumors and tumors located in the stomach appear to follow an indolent course (43,53,54). However these tumors should not be regarded as benign as GIST always carried an inherent risk of recurrence and metastasis. Pediatric GIST patients may develop metastasis despite being classified as low risk. Metastasis to local regional lymph nodes is also more common in pediatric than adults GIST (53, 54). A significant proportion of pediatric GIST is also SDH-deficient while being wild type for *KIT* and *PDGFRA*. Thus, pediatric GIST has, over the last decade, evolved as a separate entity that is distinct from adult GIST [55].

References

[1] Dei Tos AP. The reappraisal of gastrointestinal stromal tumors: from Stout to the Kit revolution. *Virchows Arch* 2003; 442: 421-428.

[2] Kindblom L-G, Remotti M E, Aldenborg F, et al. Gastrointestinal pacemaker cell tumor (GIPACT): gastrointestinal stromal tumors show phenotypic characteristics of interstitial cells of Cajal. *Am J Pathol* 1998; 152:1259-1269.

[3] Ma YY, Yu S, He XJ, et al. Involvement of c-KIT mutation in the development of gastrointestinal stromal tumors through proliferation promotion and apoptosis inhibition. *Onco Targets Ther* 2014; 7:637-43.

[4] Rubin BP, Singer S, Tsao C, et al. KIT activation is a ubiquitous feature of gastrointestinal stromal tumors. Cancer Res. 2001;61:8118–8121.

[5] Antonescu CR. Gastrointestinal stromal tumor (GIST) pathogenesis, familial GIST, and animal models. *Semin Diagn Pathol* 2006; 23(2): 63-9.

[6] Chi P, Chen Y, Zhang L, et al. ETV1 is a lineage survival factor that cooperates with KIT in gastrointestinal stromal tumours. *Nature*. 2010; 467(7317):849-53.

[7] Ran L, Sirota I, Cao Z, et al. Combined inhibition of MAP kinase and KIT signaling effectively destabilizes the ETV1 protein and synergistically suppresses GIST tumorigenesis. *Cancer Discov* 2015. pii: CD-14-0985.

[8] Birner P, Beer A, Vinatzer U, et al. MAPKAP kinase 2 overexpression influences prognosis in gastrointestinal stromal tumors and associates with copy number variations on chromosome 1 and expression of p38 MAP kinase and ETV1. *Clin Cancer Res* 2012; 18(7):1879-87.

[9] Wang Y, Marino-Enriquez A, Bennett RR, et al. Dystrophin is a tumor suppressor in human cancers with myogenic programs. *Nat Genet* 2014; 46(6):601-6.

[10] Boikos SA, Stratakis CA. The genetic landscape of gastrointestinal stromal tumor lacking KIT and PDGFRA mutations. *Endocrine* 2014; 47(2):401-8.

[11] Beadling C, Patterson J, Justusson E, et al. Gene expression of the IGF pathway family distinguishes subsets of gastrointestinal stromal tumors wild type for KIT and PDGFRA. *Cancer Med* 2013; 2:21-31.

[12] Pantaleo MA, Nannini M, Corless CL, Heinrich MC. Quadruple wild-type (WT) GIST: defining the subset of GIST that lacks abnormalities of KIT, PDGFRA, SDH, or RAS signaling pathways. *Cancer Med* 2015; 4(1):101-3.

[13] Dei Tos AP, Laurino L, Bearzi I, Messerini L, Farinati F. Gastrointestinal stromal tumors: The histology report. *Digestive and Liver Disease* 2011; 43S: S304–S309.

[14] Yamamoto H, Oda Y. Gastrointestinal stromal tumor: Recent advances in pathology and genetics. *Pathol Int* 2015; 65(1):9-18.

[15] Chandrasekhara V, Ahmad NA.EUS-guided fine needle aspiration of gastrointestinal stromal tumors: the GIST of the matter. Dig *Dis Sci* 2011; 56(6):1596-8.

[16] Miettinen M, Lasota J. Gastrointestinal stromal tumors: review on morphology, molecular pathology, prognosis, and differential diagnosis. *Arch Pathol Lab Med* 2006; 130(10):1466-78.

[17] Wong N A C S, Young R, Malcomson R D, et al. Prognostic indicators from gastrointestinal stromal tumors: a clinicopathological and immunohistochemical study of 108 resected cases of the stomach. *Histopathology* 2003; 43:118-126.

[18] Miettinen M, Sobin LH, Lasota J. Gastrointestinal stromal tumors of the stomach: a clinicopathologic, immunohistochemical, and molecular genetic study of 1765 cases with long-term follow-up. *Am J Surg Pathol* 2005; 29:52-68.

[19] Fletcher C D M, Berman J J, Corless C et al. Diagnosis of gastrointestinal stromal tumors: a consensus approach. *Hum Pathol* 2002; 33: 459-465.

[20] Miettinen M, Majidi M, Lasota J. Pathology and diagnostic criteria of gastrointestinal stromal tumors (GISTs): a review. *Eur J Cancer* 2002; 38 Suppl 5:S39-51.

[21] Trupiano JK, Stewart RE, Misick C, Appelman HD, Goldblum JR. Gastric stromal tumors: a clinicopathologic study of 77 cases with correlation of features with nonaggressive and aggressive clinical behaviors. *Am J Surg Pathol* 2002; 26(6):705-14.

[22] Patil DT, Rubin BP. Gastrointestinal stromal tumor: Advances in diagnosis and management. *Arch Pathol Lab Med* 2011; 135:1298-1310.

[23] Suster S, Sorace D, Moran C A. Gastrointestinal stromal tumors with prominent myxoid matrix. *Am J surg Pathol* 1995; 19:59-70.

[24] Suster S, Fletcher C D M. Gastrointestinal stromal tumors with prominent signet-ring cell forms. *Mod Pathol* 1996; 9:609-613.

[25] Antonescu CR, Romeo S, Zhang L, et al. Dedifferentiation in gastrointestinal stromal tumor to an anaplastic KIT-negative phenotype: a diagnostic pitfall: morphologic and molecular characterization of 8 cases occurring either de novo or after imatinib therapy. *Am J Surg Pathol* 2013; 37(3):385-92.

[26] Todaro P, Crino SF, Pallio S, Consolo P, Tuccari G. Gastrointestinal stromal tumours of the stomach: Cytological and immunocytochemical diagnostic features of two cases diagnosed by endoscopic ultrasound-guided fine needle aspiration. *Oncol Lett.* 2013; 5(6): 1862–1866.

[27] Chatzipantelis P, Salla C, Karoumpalis I, et al. Endoscopic ultrasound-guided fine needle aspiration biopsy in the diagnosis of gastrointestinal stromal tumors of the stomach. A study of 17 cases. *J Gastrointestin Liver Dis* 2008; 17(1):15-20.

[28] Gu M. Ghafari S, Nguyen PT, Lin F. Cytologic diagnosis of gastrointestinal stromal tumors of the stomach by endoscopic ultrasound-guided fine-needle aspiration biopsy: cytomorphologic and immunohistochemical study of 12 cases. *Diagn Cytopathol* 2001; 25(6):343-50.

[29] Akahoshi K, Oya M, Koga T, et al. Clinical usefulness of endoscopic ultrasound-guided fine needle aspiration for gastric subepithelial lesions smaller than 2 cm. *J Gastrointestin Liver Dis* 2014; 23(4):405-12.

[30] Newman PL, Wadden C, Fletcher CDM. Gastrointestinal stromal tumors: correlation of immunophenotype with clinicopathologic features. *J Pathol* 1991; 164:107-117.

[31] Greenson JK. Gastrointestinal stromal tumors and other mesenchymal lesions of the gut. *Mod Pathol* 2003; 16(4):366–375.
[32] Abraham SC. Distinguishing gastrointestinal stromal tumors from their mimics: an update. *Adv Anat Pathol* 2007; 14(3):178-88.
[33] Kukar M, Kapil A, Papenfuss W, Groman A, Grobmyer SR, Hochwald SN. Gastrointestinal stromal tumors (GISTs) at uncommon locations: A large population based analysis. *J Surg Oncol* 2015; 111(6):696-701.
[34] Voltaggio L, Montgomery EA. Gastrointestinal tract spindle cell lesions-just like real estate, it's all about location. *Mod Pathol* 2015; 28 Suppl 1:S47-66.
[35] Miettinen M, Sobin LH, Sarlomo-Rikala M. Immunohistochemical spectrum of GISTs at different sites and their differential diagnosis with a reference to CD117 (KIT). *Mod Pathol* 2000; 13(10):1134-42.
[36] Romeo S, Rossi S, Acosta Marín M, et al. Primary_Synovial Sarcoma (SS) of the digestive system: a molecular and clinicopathological study of fifteen cases. *Clin Sarcoma Res.* 2015; 5:7.
[37] Palmirotta R, De Marchis ML, Ludovici G, et al. Mutational analysis of gastrointestinal stromal tumors (GISTs): procedural approach for diagnostic purposes. *Cancer Genomics Proteomics* 2013; 10(3):115-23.
[38] Lasota J, Miettinen M. Clinical significance of oncogenic KIT and PDGFRA mutations in gastrointestinal stromal tumours. *Histopathology* 2008; 53(3):245-66.
[39] Heinrich M C, Corless C L, Duensing A, et al. PDGFRA activating mutations in gastrointestinal stromal tumors. *Science* 2003; 299:708-710.
[40] Lasota J, Dansonka-Mieszkowska A, Sobin LH, et al. A great majority of GISTs with PDGFRA mutations represent gastric tumors of low or no malignant potential. *Lab Invest* 2004; 84: 874-883.
[41] Bjerkehagen B, Aaberg K, Steigen SE. Do not be fooled by fancy mutations: Inflammatory fibroid polyps can harbor mutations similar to those found in GIST. *Case Rep Med* 2013; 2013:845801.
[42] Huss S, Wardelmann E, Goltz D, Binot E, Hartmann W, Merkelbach-Bruse S, Büttner R, Schildhaus HU. Activating PDGFRA mutations in inflammatory fibroid polyps occur in exons 12, 14 and 18 and are associated with tumour localization. *Histopathology* 2012; 61(1):59-68.
[43] Prakash S, Sarran L, Socci N, et al. Gastrointestinal stromal tumors in children and young adults: a clinicopathologic, molecular, and genomic study of 15 cases and review of the literature. *J Pediatr Hematol Oncol* 2005; 27:179–187.

[44] Miettinen M, Lasota J. Succinate dehydrogenase deficient gastrointestinal stromal tumors (GISTs) - a review. *Int J Biochem Cell Biol* 2014; 53:514-9.

[45] Miettinen M, Wang ZF, Sarlomo-Rikala M, Osuch C, Rutkowski P, Lasota J. Succinate dehydrogenase-deficient GISTs: a clinicopathologic, immunohistochemical, and molecular genetic study of 66 gastric GISTs with predilection to young age. *Am J Surg Pathol* 2011; 35(11):1712-21.

[46] Hostein I, Faur N, Primois C, et al. BRAF mutation status in gastrointestinal stromal tumors. *Am J Clin Pathol* 2010; 133(1):141-8.

[47] Badalamenti G, Rodolico V, Fulfaro F, et al. Gastrointestinal stromal tumors (GISTs): focus on histopathological diagnosis and biomolecular features. *Ann Oncol* 18 (Supplement 6): vi136–vi140, 2007.

[48] Dematteo RP, Gold JS, Saran L, et al. Tumor mitotic rate, size, and location independently predict recurrence after resection of primary gastrointestinal stromal tumor (GIST). Cancer 2008; 112(3):608-15.

[49] Miettinen M, Lasota J. Gastrointestinal stromal tumors: pathology and prognosis at different sites. *Semin Diagn Pathol* 2006; 23:70-83.

[50] Gronchi A. Risk stratification models and mutational analysis: keys to optimising adjuvant therapy in patients with gastrointestinal stromal tumour. *Eur J Cancer* 2013; 49(4):884-92.

[51] Bischof DA, Kim Y, Dodson R, et al. Conditional disease-free survival after surgical resection of gastrointestinal stromal tumors: A multi-institutional analysis of 502 patients. *JAMA Surg* 2015; 150(4):299-306.

[52] Joensuu H, Rutkowski P, Nishida T, et al. KIT and PDGFRA mutations and the risk of GI stromal tumor recurrence. *J Clin Oncol* 2015; 33(6):634-42.

[53] Miettinen M, Lasota J, Sobin LH. Gastrointestinal stromal tumors of the stomach in children and young adults: a clinicopathologic, immunohistochemical, and molecular genetic study of 44 cases with long-term follow-up and review of the literature. *Am J Surg Pathol* 2005; 29:1373–1381.

[54] Benesch M, Wardelmann E, Ferrari A, Brennan B, Verschuur A. Gastrointestinal stromal tumors (GIST) in children and adolescents: A comprehensive review of the current literature. *Pediatr Blood Cancer* 2009; 53(7):1171-9.

[55] Rink L, Godwin AK. Clinical and molecular characteristics of gastrointestinal stromal tumors in the pediatric and young adult population. *Curr Oncol Rep* 2009; 11(4):314-21.

In: Gastrointestinal Stromal Tumors in Adults ... ISBN: 978-1-63483-679-1
Editor: Atif A. Ahmed

Chapter 6

GASTROINTESTINAL STROMAL TUMORS IN YOUNGER PATIENTS

***Alberto S. Pappo*[1,*] *and Markku Miettinen*[2]**

[1]Solid Tumor Division, Department of Oncology,
St. Jude Children's Research Hospital,
262 Danny Thomas Place, Memphis, TN, US
[2]Laboratory of Pathology, National Cancer Institute,
Laboratory of Surgical Pathology, Bethesda, MD, US

ABSTRACT

Gastrointestinal stromal tumors (GIST) in young children have evolved as a unique entity showing striking differences from those in adults. Most GIST in young children are wild type for *KIT* and *PDGFRA* oncogenic mutations and arise by different mechanisms. They are frequently associated with tumor-specific loss of the succinate de-hydrogenase (SDH) complex function, which can be detected by immunohistochemical loss of expression or mutational testing, and are thus designated SDH-deficient GIST. SDH-deficient GIST can occur as part of the Carney-Stratakis syndrome and Carney Triad, exhibit different biologic behavior and do not follow the same prognostic parameters, like in adults. Tyrosine kinase inhibitors are not effective in treating SDH-deficient GIST. Knowledge of these biologic and behavioral differences is important in the management of young children with GIST.

* Email: alberto.pappo@stjude.org.

INTRODUCTION

Gastrointestinal stromal tumor (GIST) is the most common primary mesenchymal tumor of the gastrointestinal tract. It is derived from the neuroregulatory gastrointestinal Cajal cells or their precursors [1]. The estimated incidence ranges from 6.8 to 20 per million, however, the incidence of subclinical disease is significantly higher [1-3]. GIST most commonly affects middle-aged adults and only about 1% occur in patients under 20 year of age [4, 5]. In all, GIST affects both sexes equally and most commonly arise in the stomach (50%) and small intestine (30%) but it can occur in any segment of the GI tract with a lower frequency.

While approximately 85-90% of adult GISTs have oncogenic activating mutations of the *KIT* and *PDGFRA* oncogenes, which lead to ligand-independent kinase activation [6], most pediatric GIST arise by different mechanisms, mostly related to tumor-specific losses of the succinate dehydrogenase complex function. In the older children, pediatric GIST overlap with adult GIST including tumors driven by *KIT* mutations. While the latter group of GIST can be successfully treated with tyrosine kinase inhibitor drugs, the treatment of pediatric GIST is still evolving.

The likelihood of disease progression or dissemination in adult GIST is dependent on various factors including size of the primary tumor, mitotic rate and anatomic site. Lesions located in the stomach, those that are smaller than 5 cm and have ≤ 5 mitosis per 50 high power fields have a better prognosis [7]. The same criteria do not apply well for pediatric GIST, especially SDH-deficient GIST, which are less predictable in their behavior.

The introduction of tyrosine kinase inhibitors such as imatinib, sunitinib and regorafenib has revolutionized the treatment of KIT and PDGFR mutant GISTsand brought remarkable improvement in the outcome of these patients [8]. Unfortunately, these treatments are not typically effective in SDH-deficient GIST.

SDH DEFICIENT GIST

A significant proportion of the discoveries that will be mentioned below were facilitated through a successful collaborative effort funded by the NIH when the first Pediatric and Wild-Type GIST Clinic opened in 2008. The purpose of this clinic was to study pediatric GIST and, to date, 126 patients have attended 11 clinics. This bi-annual collaborative effort brings together patients, clinicians, researchers, and patient advocates from across the United States to better understand and characterize the clinical and genomic features of this rare disease.

The vast majority of GIST in the younger age groups are associated with tumor-specific loss of the succinate dehydrogenase (SDH) complex function, and these tumors are designated SDH-deficient GIST [9-12]. SDH-deficient status is most practically determined by immunohistochemical loss of the SDHB subunit in the tumor cells, which is a universal phenomenon among SDH-deficient tumors independent of their genetic background. Similar SDH-loss is known as the disease mechanism for 30% of extra-adrenal paragangliomas [13], and rare renal cancers [14], both of which have been observed in patients with SDH-deficient GIST.

In addition to children and young adults, SDH-deficient GIST occur in older agee groups with a lower frequency. Based on current experience, SDH-deficient GIST occur exclusively in the stomach [11, 12]. Two syndromes constitute subsets of SDH-deficient GIST: Carney-Stratakis and Carney Triad. Carney-Stratakis syndrome is characterized by the occurrence of GIST and paraganglioma in connection with a germ-line mutation in the SDH complex [15]. Carney triad includes the occurrence of GIST, pulmonary chondroma, and paraganglioma, without a mutation in the SDH-genes [16]. Due to the often asynchronous occurrence of multiple tumors in the patients, only a minority of SDH-deficient GIST fulfill the criteria of these syndromes.

Succinate dehydrogenase (SDH) is a multimeric enzyme complex located at the inner aspect of the mitochondrial membrane. It belongs to mitochondrial complex 2 and is entirely encoded by genes in the chromosomal (not mitochondrial) DNA [17]. The functions of the SDH-complex include conversion of succinate to fumarate in the Krebs cycle and the electron transport of the oxidative phosphorylation pathway. The components of the SDH-complex include SDHA, SDHB, SDHC, SDHD, and assembly factors SDHAF1 and SDHAF2. SDHA is the catalytic subunit responsible for the oxidation of succinate to fumarate. SDHB is a component in the oxidative phosphorylation via redox-events by its iron-sulphur component. SDHC and SDHD anchor SDHA and SDHB in the mitochondrial membrane [17]. SDH-deficiency leads to succinate accumulation, which affects at least two major metabolic processes outlined below [18] and is also associated with extensive genomic methylation, which is likely involved in the pathogenesis of GIST [19].

1. Succinate accumulation inhibits prolyl hydroxylases that hydroxylate and promote degradation of HIF1α, a transcriptional activator for IGF2 and VEGF. IGF2 overexpression activates IGF2 growth signaling.
2. Succinate accumulation acts as α-ketoglutarate antagonist inhibiting other α-ketoglutarate dependent dioxygenases such as the TET family of 5mc hydroxylases inhibiting histone and DNA demethylation.

Molecular Genetic Features

SDH-deficient GIST are associated with SDH-complex mutations in about 1/3 to half of patients, and most of these mutations have been germline [10, 19-21]. Most commonly mutated is SDHA (30% of all SDH-deficient GIST).. Up to half of SDH-deficient GIST are not associated with SDH complex mutations and are characterized by SDHC promoter hypermethylation leading to epigenetic silencing of the SDH-complex [22]. The germline mutations are typically associated with the loss of the other allele of the mutated SDH-subunit gene to yield silencing of one of the SDH-subunit genes according to the principles of classic tumor suppressor genes [19.20]. Mutation analysis of the entire set of SDH-subunit genes can now be performed via gene panels offered in the newer next generation sequencing systems.

Because of the significant frequency of germline SDH-mutations, analysis of consenting family members, especially siblings and parents, shopuld be undertaken with the support of genetic counseling. Based on clinical experience, occurrence of SDH-deficient GISTs in multiple siblings or child and parent seems to be uncommon suggesting that occurrence of the two hits on one SDH subunit gene must be rare.

Symptoms and Diagnosis of SDH Deficient GIST

Clinically, most of the symptomatic GIST manifest by gastrointestinal discomfort or gastrointestinal bleeding, and in this sense pediatric GIST are similar to the adult ones. However, about ⅓ of adult GIST are incidentally detected in the course of an unrelated procedure [1].

Upper GI endoscopy and endoscopy ultrasound in conjunction with esophagogastroduodeno-scopy is more accurate to define the characteristics of the lesion and to obtain a biopsy of a lesion suspicious of GIST.

Computed tomography (CT) is the recommended imaging modality. However, given the fact that most of the succinate dehydrogenase deficient GIST occur in young patients, MRI should be considered an appropriate imaging modality if the expertise and equipment are available. MRI can also be used to detect associated lesions, such as asymptomatic paragangliomas [23]. Routine scanning of the chest for metastases is not suggested in view of rarity of lung metastases, and PET should not be routinely used.

PATHOLOGY OF SDH-DEFICIENT GIST

SDH-deficient GIST are often histologically distinctive. They often involve the gastric wall in a multinodular manner leading strands of pre-existing smooth muscle between the nodules (Figure 1 A). This is commonly referred to as "plexiform growth pattern". Tumor cells have usually epithelioid (non-spindled) morphology (Figure 1 B), but some cases have a mixture of epithelioid and spindle cells or composed entirely of spindled cells. Substantial nuclear pleomorphism may occur in this group. Features that are nearly exclusive to SDH-deficient GIST are lymphovascular invasion (up to half of cases), and lymph node metastases in 10% of cases (Figure 1 C). Omental, other intra-abdominal, and liver metastases occur as seen in adult GIST. In many cases, metastasis is delayed, and metastases have been seen in 40 years after the primary tumor [11].

Immunohistochemically SDH-deficient GIST are characterized by loss of the SDHB, which is observed as lack of the otherwise ubiquitous SDHB expression in the tumor cells, while expression is maintained in the stromal cells and other non-neoplastic elements (Figure 1 D). Only those SDH-deficient GIST that are based on SDHA-mutations are SDHA negative. All SDH-deficient GIST are equally KIT-positive as are KIT/PDGFRA mutant GIST. A majority of them are also positive for CD34.

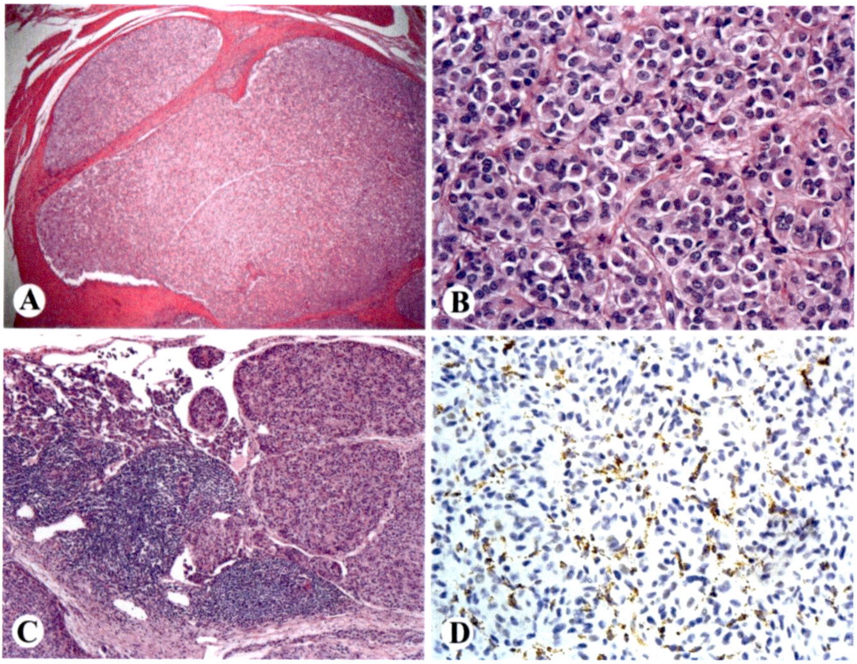

Figure 1. Histologic features of an SDH-deficient GIST. A. Multinodular gastric wall involvement with spared streaks of gastric smooth muscle is typical. B. Most cases show distinctly epithelioid cytology. C. Lymph node metastases occur only in SDH-deficient GISTs. D. SDH-deficient status can be ascertained by SDHB-immunohistochemistry, which shows loss of this generally ubiquitous protein, with expression retained in non-neoplastic elements such as vascular septa.

TREATMENT

Surgery is the primary mode of therapy for patients with any GIST. Limited operation such as laparoscopic wedge resection is a consideration for small and solitary lesions. Open surgery is generally required for large or multifocal tumors, which may necessitate antrectomy, or subtotal or even total gastrectomy. Because lymph nodes can be involved, attention to perigastric regional nodes and peritoneal nodules, is advisable. Aggressive operations that will leave macroscopic disease should be avoided unless they relieve impending problems, such as hemorrhage or obstruction [24].

SDH-deficient GIST are usually not sensitive to tyrosine kinase inhibitor drugs, neither as a first line inhibitor nor as a second line. New agents such as angiogenesis inhibitors (vandetanib), IGF1R inhibitors (OSI-906) or demethylating agents are either currently being investigated or will be investigated in the near future.

Postoperative surveillance has not been well established in this group of tumors, but it is suggested that chest x-rays and MRI or CT scans of the abdomen be done every 3 months for 1 year and every 6 months thereafter as recently suggested. Initial assessment of tumor growth can be done with imaging at initial 6 week intervals, followed by physical examinations, labs, chest radiograph, and MRI of the abdomen and pelvis at 3 month intervals for 24 months, followed by 6 month interval for 24 months, and then yearly thereafter [24].

KIT/PDGFRA Mutant GISTs in Younger Age Groups

KIT/PDGFRA mutant GIST are very rare in the pediatric age group but begin to occur in the late teen years. These GIST are not restricted to stomach and often occur in the small intestine and less commonly in other sites such as the rectum. KIT germline mutation-related familial GIST only rarely clinically manifest at a young age, but may occur from the 2nd decade. The clinical features and management of KIT mutant GIST are essentially similar to adult KIT/PDGFRA mutant GIST and frequently involve tyrosine kinase inhibitors [25, 26].

Neurofibromatosis 1-Associated GIST

Approximately 1-2% of GIST arise in patients with neurofibromatosis type 1. These tumors more commonly affect females and occur at a median age of 49 years. Most GISTs in these patients are small, multifocal, have a low mitotic rate, have spindle cell morphology and arise in the small intestine. NF1-associated GIST express KIT by immunohistochemistry and lack KIT and PDFGR mutations [27]. Patients with NF1 and GIST commonly present with gastrointestinal bleeding and have a favorable clinical outcome in the majority of cases. The pathogenesis of NF1-associated GIST seems to be associated with the RAS-signaling activation as a consequence of loss of NF1-function [28].

BRAF Mutant GIST

A small number of KIT/PDGFRA wild type GIST have been reported to harbor a BRAF V600E mutation more often seen in melanoma and colon cancer, among others. These GIST more commonly affect females, are mainly localized in the small intestine, often have spindle cell or mixed morphology and affect adults in their 5th and 6th decade of life [29, 30]. A recent report suggests that these tumors may besensitive to the selective BRAF inhibitor dabrafenib [31].

In addition to the above mentioned category, there is a group of "quadruple wild-type" GISTs that lack pathogenic mutations in the genes KIT, PDGFRA, SDHX, BRAF, and RAS but show a unique expression profile characterized by overexpression of the NTRK2 and ERG oncogenes [32].

References

[1] Miettinen M, Lasota J: Gastrointestinal stromal tumors. *Gastroenterol Clin North Am* 2013; 42:399-415.

[2] Perez EA, Livingstone AS, Franceschi D, et al: Current incidence and outcomes of gastrointestinal mesenchymal tumors including gastrointestinal stromal tumors. *J Am Coll Surg* 2006; 202:623-9.

[3] Agaimy A, Wunsch PH, Hofstaedter F, et al: Minute gastric sclerosing stromal tumors (GIST tumorlets) are common in adults and frequently show c-KIT mutations. *Am J Surg Pathol* 2007; 31:113-20.

[4] Mastrangelo G, Coindre JM, Ducimetiere F, et al: Incidence of soft tissue sarcoma and beyond: a population-based prospective study in 3 European regions. *Cancer* 2012; 118:5339-48.

[5] Prakash S, Sarran L, Socci N, et al: Gastrointestinal stromal tumors in children and young adults: a clinicopathologic, molecular, and genomic study of 15 cases and review of the literature. *J Pediatr Hematol Oncol* 2005; 27:179-87.

[6] Corless CL, Barnett CM, Heinrich MC: Gastrointestinal stromal tumours: origin and molecular oncology. Nature reviews. *Cancer* 2011; 11:865-78.

[7] Miettinen M, Lasota J: Gastrointestinal stromal tumors: review on morphology, molecular pathology, prognosis, and differential diagnosis. *Arch Pathol Lab Med* 2006; 130:1466-78.

[8] Serrano C, George S: Recent advances in the treatment of gastrointestinal stromal tumors. *Ther Adv Med Oncol* 2014; 6:115-27.

[9] Gill AJ, Chou A, Vilain R, et al. Immunohistochemistry for SDHB divides gastrointestinal stromal tumors (GISTs) into 2 distinct types. *Am J Surg Pathol* 2010; 34:636-44.

[10] Janeway KA, Kim SY, Lodish M, et al: Defects in succinate dehydrogenase in gastrointestinal stromal tumors lacking KIT and PDGFRA mutations. *Proc Natl Acad Sci USA;* 2011; 108:314-8.

[11] Miettinen M, Wang ZF, Sarlomo-Rikala M, et al: Succinate dehydrogenase-deficient GISTs: a clinicopathologic, immune-histochemical, and molecular genetic study of 66 gastric GISTs with predilection to young age. *Am J Surg Pathol* 2011; 35:1712-21.

[12] Miettinen M, Lasota J: Succinate dehydrogenase deficient gastrointestinal stromal tumors (Gists) - A review. *Int J Biochem Cell Biol* 2014; 53:514-9.

[13] van Nederveen FH, Gaal J, Favier J, et al An immunohistochemical procedure to detect patients with paraganglioma and phaeochromocytoma with germline SDHB, SDHC, or SDHD gene mutations: a retrospective and prospective analysis. *Lancet Oncol* 2009; 10:764-771.

[14] Gill AJ, Hes O, Papathomas T, et al. Succinate dehydrogenase (SDH)-deficient renal carcinoma: A morphologically distinct entity: A clinicopathologic series of 36 tumors from 27 patients. *Am J Surg Pathol* 2014; 38(12):1588-602.

[15] Pasini B, McWhinney SR, Bei T, et al: Clinical and molecular genetics of patients with the Carney-Stratakis syndrome and germline mutations of the genes coding for the succinate dehydrogenase subunits SDHB, SDHC, and SDHD. *Eur J Hum Genet* 2008; 16:79-88.

[16] Carney JA, Sheps SG, Go VL, et al: The triad of gastric leiomyosarcoma, functioning extra-adrenal paraganglioma and pulmonary chondroma. *N Engl J Med.* 1977; 296:1517-8.

[17] Rutter J, Winge DR, Schiffman JD. Succinate dehydrogenase - Assembly, regulation and role in human disease. *Mitochondrion* 2010; 10:393-401.

[18] Boikos SA, Stratakis CA: The genetic landscape of gastrointestinal stromal tumor lacking KIT and PDGFRA mutations. *Endocrine* 2014; 47(2):401-8.

[19] Killian JK, Kim SY, Miettinen M, et al: Succinate dehydrogenase mutation underlies global epigenomic divergence in gastrointestinal stromal tumor. *Cancer Discov* 2013; 3(6):648-57.

[20] Miettinen M, Killian JK, Wang ZF, et al. Immunohistochemical loss of succinate dehydrogenase subunit A (SDHA) in gastrointestinal stromal tumors (GISTs) signals SDHA germline mutation. *Am J Surg Pathol* 2013; 37:234-240.

[21] Pantaleo MA, Astolfi A, Urbini M, et al. Analysis of all subunits, SDHA, SDHB, SDHC, SDHD, of the succinate dehydrogenase complex in KIT/PDGFRA wild-type GIST. *Eur J Hum Genet* 2014; 22:32-39.

[22] Killian JK, Miettinen M, Walker RL, et al. Recurrent epimutation of SDHC in gastrointestinal stromal tumors. *Sci Transl Med* 2014; 6(268):268ra177.

[23] Jasperson KW, Kohlmann W, Gammon A, et al. Role of rapid sequence whole-body MRI screening in SDH-associated hereditary paraganglioma families. *Fam Cancer* 2014; 13:257-65.

[24] Pappo AS, Janeway KA: Pediatric gastrointestinal stromal tumors. *Hematol Oncol Clin North Am* 2009; 23:15-34, vii.

[25] Agaram NP, Laquaglia MP, Ustun B, et al. Molecular characterization of pediatric gastrointestinal stromal tumors. *Clin Cancer Res* 2008; 14:3204-3215.

[26] 26. Kang G, Park YS, Jung ES, et al. Gastrointestinal stromal tumors in children and young adults: a clinicopathologic and molecular genetic study of 22 Korean cases. *APMIS* 2013; 121:938-944.

[27] Miettinen M, Fetsch JF, Sobin LH, et al: Gastrointestinal stromal tumors in patients with neurofibromatosis 1: a clinicopathologic and molecular genetic study of 45 cases. *Am J Surg Pathol* 2006; 30:90-6.

[28] Maertens O, Prenen H, Debiec-Rychter M, et al. Molecular pathogenesis of multiple gastrointestinal stromal tumors in NF1 patients. *Hum Mol Genet* 2006; 15:1015-1023.

[29] Hostein I, Faur N, Primois C, et al: BRAF mutation status in gastrointestinal stromal tumors. *Am J Clin Pathol* 2010; 133:141-8.

[30] Daniels M, Lurkin I, Pauli R, et al: Spectrum of KIT/PDGFRA/BRAF mutations and Phosphatidylinositol-3-Kinase pathway gene alterations in gastrointestinal stromal tumors (GIST). *Cancer Lett* 2011; 312:43-54.

[31] Falchook GS, Trent JC, Heinrich MC, et al: BRAF mutant gastrointestinal stromal tumor: first report of regression with BRAF inhibitor dabrafenib (GSK2118436) and whole exomic sequencing for analysis of acquired resistance. *Oncotarget* 2013; 4:310-5.

[32] Nannini M, Astolfi A, Urbini M, et al. Integrated genomic study of quadruple-WT GIST (KIT/PDGFRA/SDH/RAS pathway wild-type GIST). *BMC Cancer* 2014; 14:685.

In: Gastrointestinal Stromal Tumors in Adults ... ISBN: 978-1-63483-679-1
Editor: Atif A. Ahmed

Chapter 7

MEDICAL TREATMENT OF GIST AND HEALTHCARE COSTS

***Deepa Susan Phillip*[1], *Bhawna Sirohi*[2,*] *and Shailesh V. Shrikhande*[3]**
[1]Department of Medical Oncology, Tata Memorial Centre, Mumbai
[2]Department of Medical Oncology Mazumdar Shaw Cancer Centre, Narayana Health, Bangalore
[3]Department of GI and HPB surgery, Tata Memorial Centre, Mumbai, India

ABSTRACT

Gastrointestinal stromal tumours (GISTs) are the most common mesenchymal tumours with a unique driver mutation in c-kit which makes it amenable to targeted treatment with tyrosine kinase inhibitor imatinib. Surgery followed by adjuvant treatment with imatinib for three years is the standard of care in high risk tumours. Neoadjuvant imatinib is increasingly being used for locally advanced unresectable tumours at presentation. For patients with advanced GIST, the FDA has approved three drugs – imatinib, sunitinib and regorafenib. In this review we focus on the use of various treatment modalities in patients with GIST and also discuss the cost-effectiveness and relevance to their use of these in India,

* Address for correspondence: Dr Bhawna Sirohi. Consultant Medical Oncologist and Head of Medical Oncology, Mazumdar Shaw Cancer Centre, Narayana Health, Bangalore. Tel: 0091 9538145698; Email: bhawna.sirohi13@gmail.com.

a developing country. Imatinib has quite a few generic versions available for use in India but there are currently no generic drugs available for sunitinib and regorafenib.

INTRODUCTION

Gastrointestinal stromal tumours (GISTs) are the most common mesenchymal tumours of the gastrointestinal tract [1], derived from the Interstitial cells of Cajal. These tumours have distinct tumour biology and inherent chemoresistance capabilities. The discovery by Hirota and colleagues [2] in 1998 of c-*KIT* mutation and intracellular signalling pathway was a landmark in the determination of aetiology of a disease at molecular level. Over the last two decades, KIT-directed therapy has changed the landscape of treatment. In this chapter, we give an overview on the medical management of GIST, with emphasis on the problems and challenges unique to the developing world.

NEO-ADJUVANT THERAPY

The use of neoadjuvant therapy with Imatinib in localized, non metastatic GIST is a decision that is to be taken in a multi-disciplinary joint clinic on an individual case to case basis. It may be planned in patients with potentially resectable but very large tumours where the risk of rupture or bleeding during surgery is high and R0 resection (i.e., complete resection with remission) may be unlikely, in those with tumours that are poorly located making R0 resection with an extensive surgery and functional deficit (e.g., rectal GIST) risky, if surgery needs to be delayed for other medical indications, in the case of unresectable locally advanced GIST for downstaging, and to decrease surgical morbidity/mortality. The standard practice is to give Imatinib at a dose of 400mg daily, in accordance with the National Comprehensive Cancer Network (NCCN), the European Society of Medical Oncology (ESMO) and Indian Council of Medical Research (ICMR) guidelines [3-6]. The optimal duration of pre-operative therapy is undefined, but usually it is continued until a maximal response is achieved (approximately 6-12 months) [7].

LOCALIZED GIST

Surgery is the primary therapeutic modality in localized resectable tumours followed by surveillance. R0 resections are usually possible in about 85% of patients but even in this patient group, 50% develop recurrence or metastasis in the absence of adjuvant therapy within a median time of 2 yrs after surgery in the high risk group [8, 9]. It would not be clinically indicated, practically feasible or cost effective to offer adjuvant therapy to all patients. Hence patients are risk stratified post operatively and patients with high risk of recurrence (i.e., tumour size >10 cm and any mitotic index, any tumour size and mitotic index >10, tumour size 5 cm and mitotic index >5, tumour size ≤5 cm and mitotic index >5 in a non-gastric site, tumour size 5.1-10 cm and mitotic index ≤5 in non-gastric site, and any tumour size and any mitotic index in the presence of tumour rupture) should be offered Imatinib. The optimal duration of Imatinib therapy in high risk GIST in the adjuvant setting is still a matter of ongoing debate with more studies in progress but current standard of care is to offer three years of adjuvant therapy. The phase III SSGXVIII/AIO study [10] showed a significantly better recurrence free survival (RFS) at 5 yrs of 66% vs. 48% and a significant improvement in overall survival (OS) at 5yrs of 92% vs. 82%, in patients receiving 3 years of adjuvant Imatinib compared with 1 year of therapy. Based on these results, the NCCN and ICMR guidelines recommend treatment with adjuvant Imatinib for at least 36 months for patients with high-risk GIST [3, 11].

The concerning fact in both arms of the above study is that there were increased recurrences after discontinuation of therapy at 3yrs, raising serious concerns about need for continuous kinase suppression in the adjuvant setting. This concern will be answered in future trials, like PERSIST-5, on prolonging the duration of therapy to 5yrs. In an ideal case scenario, before starting adjuvant therapy, mutational analysis is crucial so that Imatinib resistant mutations, e.g., PDGFRA D-842V mutation, may not be given Imatinib, as it would have no benefit and so would not be cost effective. Furthermore, GIST with KIT exon 9 mutation may be offered higher dose of Imatinib, i.e., 800mg, so that drug resistance and disease progression could be avoided [12, 13].

Cost-Effectiveness

In a study conducted by Sanon et al. [14], that assessed the cost-effectiveness (CE) of treating patients with 3 years versus 1 year of adjuvant

Imatinib from a US payer's perspective, a Markov model was developed to predict GIST recurrence and treatment costs, expected costs and quality-adjusted life years (QALYs). With the limitations of the simulation models, the study concluded that treating surgically resected *KIT*+ GIST patients with 3 years of Imatinib would result in improved quality-adjusted survival (8.53 vs 7.18) and was cost effective in 100% of the simulations.

METASTATIC DISEASE

First-Line Setting

Imatinib is the standard of care in the first line therapy for patients with metastatic GIST. The standard dose of Imatinib administered is 400mg daily [15-16]. In patients harbouring exon 9 *KIT* mutations a higher dose of 800mg daily of Imatinib is recommended. Wozniac et al. have shown that patients on 800 mg dose had improvement in progression-free survival (PFS) (6 vs. 19 months; P = 0.017) and showed tendency to impact OS (28 vs. 35 months, P = 0.15) [16]. The EORTC-ISG-AGITG 62005 trial also showed that patients with *KIT* exon 9 mutations had lower response to Imatinib (34% vs. 68% for *KIT* exon 11) that translated into a shorter PFS [15]. Also patients with *KIT* exon 9 mutation had improved PFS with higher (800 mg/ day) dose of Imatinib (median PFS of 18 vs. 6 months). In view of above data, NCCN and ESMO recommend a dose of 800mg/day for patients harbouring *KIT* exon 9 mutation [3-6].

Imatinib therapy is to be continued indefinitely until progression or unacceptable side effects occur. It has been shown in some studies that there is rapid progression of disease with treatment interruption and discontinuation [17]. The BFR14 randomized phase III study conducted by the French Sarcoma Group have studied the impact of interrupting treatment after 1 year, 3 years, or 5 years of 400mg of imatinib in patients with advanced GIST [17]. Discontinuation of drug after 1 year resulted in increased disease progression of 81% compared to 31% in the continuation group. Discontinuation at 3yrs also affected the PFS with 80% versus 16% in the interruption arm. Treatment interruption after 5 years of imatinib also resulted in rapid disease progression in 45% as opposed to no patients progressing when included in the continuation arm. Updated results of 2011 show that the median PFS in 1-yr, 3-yr, 5-yr and continuation groups were 7, 9, 13 and 29 months respectively. These studies clearly show that continued uninterrupted *KIT* kinase blockade is mandatory in all patients of metastatic GIST unless they develop significant toxicity [18-23].

Cost-Effectiveness

In a review of pharmacoeconomic studies conducted by Blanke et al. from Vancouver, to determine the CE of first and second-line therapies in GIST, six studies were identified, including three analyses of first-line imatinib and three analyses of second -line sunitinib. Despite study limitations, studies of first-line imatinib showed that imatinib was CE in advanced, metastatic GIST. The limitations of these pharmacoeconomic studies included the use of survival as endpoint and required projections of outcomes beyond available data, and diversity in the countries of origin/currency/patient demographics/health care systems [24].

Second-Line and Beyond Setting

If patients progress on imatinib, the standard approach is to increase the dose from 400 mg to 800 mg daily [25]. In the EORTC trial, crossover of patients to dose escalated arm translated to improvement in survival [26]. The NCCN guidelines recommend the use of Sunitinib as second line therapy for advanced GIST at the dosage schedule of 50 mg per day on a schedule of four weeks on and 2 weeks off, or a continuous daily dose of 37.5 mg per day, at the physician's discretion [27]. The option of Sunitinib therapy for GIST became a reality after it received FDA approval in 2006 for the treatment of advanced Imatinib -resistant GIST or for patients that are Imatinib-intolerant [28].

After failing on Sunitinib, patients with metastatic GIST can be considered for third-line treatment with regorafenib [29]. Regorafenib was approved in February 2013 for locally advanced, unresectable GISTs that no longer responded to Imatinib or Sunitinib. In the phase III randomised GRID trial of 199 patients with metastatic or unresectable GIST, patients were randomized to either regorafenib (160 mg daily for 3 weeks followed by a 1-week break) or placebo and this showed a significant improvement in PFS with Regorafenib [4.8 vs. 0.9months].

In patients who have exhausted all available therapies or in whom second line therapies are not feasible to explore, NCCN guidelines recommend a re-challenge or continuation of Imatinib at and beyond disease progression, even if they have been treated with Imatinib in first line setting. A clinical trial exploring this hypothesis (Rechallenge of Imatinib in GIST Having No Effective Treatment, or RIGHT) from Korea[30] has shown that rechallenge with Imatinib significantly improves PFS and disease control rates in patients with advanced GIST after failure of Imatinib and Sunitinib most probably by continued kinase blockade in the disease clones retaining tyrosine kinase inhibitor (TKI) sensitivity. However the resistant clones continue to have progression leading to short lives despite significant benefit with this approach.

HEALTH CARE CHALLENGES

All of the above approaches apply to Indian patients and patients in other third world countries. Healthcare is funded for a minority of patients via third party insurance and majority of patients have to self-pay. The patient support programmes like GIPAP (http://www.themaxfoundation.org/gipap/) for Gleevec play a useful role for patients who are below poverty line or who satisfy the criteria for inclusion into the program. We need to strike a balance between the rising costs of expensive new anticancer agents, diagnostic imaging, and more broadly of managing GIST as a chronic disease. The cost of branded Imatinib 400mg (Gleevec) in India is approximately Rs. 100,000/- per month and about Rs. 10000-Rs 12000/- per month for Generic brands of Imatinib (there are currently 10 generic versions available).

Global communication is the need of the hour to bring together patient advocacy groups from around the world to share their ideas and experiences which would provide both clinical and psychological benefits. Inefficient clinical trials would lead to waste of money and time in rare tumours. These resources need to be better utilised to optimise care in developing countries. Another unique problem of India is the availability of many generic drugs with lack of quality control and without proper bioequivalence studies. Bureaucratic hurdles may be there on the way to patient care and hence patient advocates may have to be more vocal regarding costs and substandard care. Recently there has been increasing interest in the issue of pharmacokinetics of Imatinib and plasma drug level monitoring. This might lead to very useful results of correlation with clinical outcomes and drug resistance.

With life-long or up to 3 years of adjuvant imatinib recommendations, there is the issue of drug compliance and adherence to therapy. Despite counselling and awareness about the disease, there are always practical issues of adherence with oral medications when they need to be taken for years and sometimes for life. For quite a few patients who are feeling absolutely fine post surgery or being in remission from advanced disease, the travel to hospital means loss of labour for a day and adhering to medication is no longer a priority. For many patients we see in the clinic, cancer treatment takes a backseat in their life, until disease recurrence and drug resistance emerge.

There has to be a sense of urgency in the management of rare cancers like GIST which are potentially curable, easily treatable and demand continued care like other chronic diseases. In developing countries, however, infectious diseases get priority before cancer among the health policy makers. So, strategic partnerships are needed to promote clinical advocacy in these diseases.

GIST Patient Support Groups and Assistance Programs

NCCN Patient Portal

It provides valuable information to patients and caregivers regarding the nature of disease, treatment options, and latest advances.

The MAX Foundation and the GIPAP Program

The Max Foundation is a US-based international non-profit dedicated to assisting underprivileged patients. The MAX Foundation administers Novartis' Glivec International Patient Assistant Program (GIPAP), and assists with treatment access. Through a highly dedicated team of local advocates based in targeted countries including India, families receive personalized support and care.

First Resource

This is a patient assistance programme for obtaining easy access to Sutent, sponsored by Pfizer.

Emerging Med

This is a Clinical Trial Matching Service that is available to GIST Support international members. It is a simple and confidential way to obtain information on current clinical trials in GIST.

GIST Cancer Awareness Foundation

It aims to support GIST patients and their families through established community support groups; increase public awareness of GIST using private and public media tools; and to raise funds for research grants.

Global Alliance and Patient Advocacy Groups

Patient advocacy groups such as the Rarer Cancers Forum UK and Sarcoma Patients EuroNet (SPAEN) demonstrate how a big collective voice offers better services from providers, more mutual support, more of cost effective multinational research projects on rarer diseases, improved access to clinical trials and louder voice to campaign at policy making level, where cancer [especially the rare cancers] takes a hind seat behind other health priorities like infections.

THE FUTURE

Mutational analysis of tumours is needed upfront to exclude insensitive mutations/Exon 9 *KIT* mutation prior to therapy so that we can avoid wastage of valuable time before optimal surgery due to non-response/progression on Imatinib [11]. PET Scans are currently being investigated as an early surrogate marker of in vivo Imatinib sensitivity [31].

REFERENCES

[1] Miettinen M, Lasota J. Gastrointestinal stromal tumours: pathology and prognosis at different sites. *Semin Diagn Pathol* 2006; 23(2):70-83.

[2] Hirota S, Isozaki K, Moriyama Y, et al. Gain-of-function mutations of c-kit in human gastrointestinal stromal tumors. *Science* 1998; 279(5350):577-80.

[3] Shrikhande SV, Sirohi B, Barretto G, et al. ICMR consensus on management of gastrointestinal stromal tumors. *Indian J Med Paediatr Oncol* 2014; 35(4):244-8.

[4] National Comprehensive Cancer Network (NCCN) guidelines. Available from: http://www.nccn.org.

[5] Demetri GD, Benjamin RS, Blanke CD, et al. NCCN Task Force report: management of patients with gastrointestinal stromal tumor (GIST)--update of the NCCN clinical practice guidelines. *J Natl Compr Canc Netw* 2007; 5 (Suppl 2): S1-29; quiz S30.
[6] ESMO/European Sarcoma Network Working Group. Gastrointestinal stromal tumors: ESMO Clinical Practice Guidelines for diagnosis, treatment and follow-up. *Ann Oncol* 2012; 23 Suppl 7:vii49-55.
[7] Shrikhande SV, Marda SS, Suradkar K, et al. Gastrointestinal stromal tumors: Case series of 29 patients defining the role of imatinib prior to surgery. *World J Surg* 2012; 36:864-71.
[8] Beham AW, Schaefer IM, Schüler P, Cameron S, Ghadimi BM. Gastrointestinal stromal tumors. *Int J Colorectal Dis* 2012; 27: 689-700.
[9] Stamatakos M, Douzinas E, Stefanaki C, et al. Gastrointestinal stromal tumor. *World J Surg Oncol* 2009; 7: 61.
[10] Joensuu H, Eriksson M, Sundby Hall K, et al. One vs three years of adjuvant imatinib for operable gastrointestinal stromal tumor: a randomized trial. *JAMA*. 2012; 307(12):1265-72.
[11] Jiang WZ, Guan GX, Lu HS, et al. Adjuvant imatinib treatment after R0 resection for patients with high-risk gastrointestinal stromal tumors: A median follow-up of 44 months. *J Surg Oncol* 2011;104: 760–764.
[12] Debiec-Rychter M, Sciot R, Le Cesne A, et al. KIT mutations and dose selection for imatinib in patients with advanced gastrointestinal stromal tumours. *Eur J Cancer* 2006; 42 (8): 1093-103.
[13] Gastrointestinal Stromal Tumor Meta-Analysis Group (MetaGIST). Comparison of two doses of imatinib for the treatment of unresectable or metastatic gastrointestinal stromal tumors: A meta-analysis of 1,640 patients. *J Clin Oncol* 2010; 28:1247-53.
[14] Sanon M, Taylor D, Parthan A, Coombs J, Paolantonio M, Sasane M. Cost-effectiveness of 3-years of adjuvant imatinib in gastrointestinal stromal tumors (GIST) in the United States. *J Med Econ* 2013; 16(1):150-159.
[15] Gastrointestinal Stromal Tumor Meta-analysis Group. Comparison of two doses of imatinib for the treatment of unresectable or metastatic gastrointestinal stromal tumors (GIST): A meta-analyis based on 1,640 patients. *J Clin Oncol* 2007; 25 (18 Suppl.):10004 [ASCO annual meeting abstract]
[16] Wozniak A, Floris G, Debiec-Rychter M, Sciot R, Schöffski P. Implications of mutational analysis for the management of patients with

gastrointestinal stromal tumors and the application of targeted therapies. *Cancer Invest* 2010; 28:839-48.

[17] Blay JY, Le CA, Ray-Coquard I, et al. Prospective multicentric randomized Phase III study of imatinib in patients with advanced gastrointestinal stromal tumors comparing interruption versus continuation of treatment beyond 1 year: The French Sarcoma Group. *J Clin Oncol* 2007; 25:1107-13.

[18] Demetri GD, von Mehren M, Blanke CD, et al. Efficacy and safety of imatinib mesylate in advanced gastrointestinal stromal tumors. *N Engl J Med* 2002; 347:472-80.

[19] Blanke CD, Demetri GD, von Mehren M, et al. Long-term results from a randomized phase II trial of standard- versus higher-dose imatinib mesylate for patients with unresectable or metastatic gastrointestinal stromal tumors expressing KIT. *J Clin Oncol* 2008; 26: 620–625.

[20] Blanke CD, Rankin C, Demetri GD, et al. Phase III randomized, intergroup trial assessing imatinib mesylate at two dose levels in patients with unresectable or metastatic gastrointestinal stromal tumors expressing the kit receptor tyrosine kinase: S0033. *J Clin Oncol* 2008; 26:626–632.

[21] Verweij J, Casali PG, Zalcberg J, et al. Progression-free survival in gastrointestinal stromal tumors with high-dose imatininb: randomized trial. *Lancet* 2004; 364: 1127–1134.

[22] Reichardt P. Optimal use of targeted agents for advanced gastrointestinal stromal tumours. *Oncology* 2010; 78(2):130-40.

[23] Le Cesne A, Ray-Coquard I, Bui BN, et al. Discontinuation of imatinib in patients with advanced gastrointestinal stromal tumors after 3 years of treatment: an open label multicentre randomised phase 3 trial. *Lancet Oncol* 2010; 11: 942–949.

[24] Blanke CD, Huse DM. Cost effectiveness of tyrosine kinase inhibitor therapy in metastatic gastrointestinal stromal tumors. *J Med Econ* 2010; 13(4):681-90.

[25] Blanke CD, Rankin C, Demetri GD, et al. Phase III randomized, intergroup trial assessing imatinib mesylate at two dose levels in patients with unresectable or metastatic gastrointestinal stromal tumors expressing the kit receptor tyrosine kinase: S0033. *J Clin Oncol* 2008; 26:626-32.

[26] Zalcberg JR, Verweij J, Casali PG, et al. Outcome of patients with advanced gastro-intestinal stromal tumours crossing over to a daily

imatinib dose of 800 mg after progression on 400 mg. *Eur J Cancer* 2005;41:1751-7.

[27] Demetri GD, van Oosterom AT, Garrett CR et al. Efficacy and safety of sunitinib in patients with advanced gastrointestinal stromal tumor after failure of imatinib: a randomised controlled trial. *Lancet* 2006; 368: 1329–1338.

[28] George S, Blay JY, Casali PG, et al. Clinical evaluation of continuous daily dosing of sunitinib malate in patients with advanced gastrointestinal stromal tumour after imatinib failure. *Eur J Cancer* 2009; 45:1959-68.

[29] Demetri GD, Reichardt P, Kang YK et al. Efficacy and safety of regorafenib for advanced gastrointestinal stromal tumours after failure of imatinib and sunitinib (GRID): an international, multicentre, randomised, placebo-controlled, phase 3 trial. *Lancet* 2013; 381:295–302.

[30] Kang YK, Ryu MH, Yoo C et al. Resumption of imatinib to control metastatic or unresectable gastrointestinal stromal tumours after failure of imatinib and sunitinib (RIGHT): a randomised, placebo-controlled, phase 3 trial. *Lancet Oncol* 2013; 14: 1175–1182.

[31] Gayed I, Vu T, Iyer R, et al. The role of 18F-FDG PET in staging and early prediction of response to therapy of recurrent gastrointestinal stromal tumors. *J Nucl Med* 45 (1): 17-21, 2004.

In: Gastrointestinal Stromal Tumors in Adults … ISBN: 978-1-63483-679-1
Editor: Atif A. Ahmed

Chapter 8

FUTURE RESEARCH DIRECTIONS

Gabriel Minarik*

Comenius University in Bratislava Faculty of Medicine,
Institute of Molecular Biomedicine, Bratislava, Slovakia

ABSTRACT

Numerous advances have been made in the last decade in the diagnosis, prognosis and treatment of gastrointestinal stromal tumor (GIST) that transformed our understanding of GIST as a well-defined clinicopathologic and molecular entity. GIST represents an example of the successful translation of results of basic molecular research to the daily clinical routine and integration of molecular data with its clinico-morphological characteristics. Despite these great achievements, research is still pending in numerous areas, particularly in the subtypes of GIST that are negative for CD117 expression, carry no mutations in *KIT* or *PDGFRa* genes and those tumors that develop resistance to the ongoing therapy with one of the tyrosine kinase inhibitors. Patients could benefit from future research on the identification of novel biomarkers with diagnostic and therapeutical value, discovery of novel genes and mutations associated with initiation and progression of the disease, novel therapeutics discoveries and advances in GIST therapy, and implementation of novel methods for disease detection and therapy monitoring.

* Email: gabriel.minarik@gmail.com.

Introduction

Several ground-breaking milestones were achieved in the past 10 years in the diagnosis, prognosis and treatment of gastrointestinal stromal tumor (GIST). GIST has changed from an incurable oncological disease with short median overall survival (~12 months) to a well defined clinicopathologic entity with long median overall survival (>5 years) [1]. This progress was associated with three important discoveries – the identification of CD117 as a sensitive and specific marker of GISTs [2]; the identification of *KIT* and *PDGFRa* activating oncogenic mutations [3, 4] and the successful application of targeted therapy with tyrosine kinase inhibitors (TKI), i.e., imatinib mesylate (Glivec®, formerly STI571) to patients with highly metastatic disease [5]. Nowadays GIST represents the typical example of the successful translation of results of basic molecular research to the daily clinical routine, as the diagnosis, prognosis and therapy of the disease is managed with use of integration of the clinico-morphological characteristics and the molecular data [6].

In spite of these great successes, problems still exist in the diagnosis, prognosis and therapy of GIST particularly in the subtypes of GIST that are negative for CD117 expression, carry no mutations in *KIT* or *PDGFRa* genes or develop resistance to the ongoing therapy with one of the currently available TKIs. These patients could benefit from future research focusing on:

1. Identification of novel biomarkers with diagnostic, prognostic and therapeutical values;
2. Discovery of novel genes and mutations associated with initiation and progression of the disease;
3. Novel therapeutics discoveries and advances in GIST therapy; and
4. Implementation of novel methods for disease detection and therapy monitoring.

1. Identification of Novel Biomarkers with Diagnostic and Prognostic Value

CD117 expression and presence of *KIT* or *PDGFRa* activating mutations are the current routinely used biomarkers for GIST diagnosis that are implemented as results of the ongoing research in this field. In 2009, DOG1 expression was confirmed as novel diagnostic biomarker by validation on large cohort of samples with similar sensitivity and specificity as CD117 [7]. In 2012, SDHB expression deficiency was recorded as mutually exclusive finding in significant proportion of so called "wild-type" GISTs, in which no other diagnostic biomarker could be used [8]. In a recent study, analysis of "wild type" GISTs, with respect to the expression of IGF1R, neural markers, INSR, KIT, CD34, IGF1, IGF2 and SDHB, showed that, based on differences of expression of these biomarkers, three different subgroups of GIST in adult patients could be identified. While in pediatric samples only one pattern was recorded. These findings confirmed the high level of heterogeneity of "wild type" GISTs and that these different subgroups could represent distinct clinical entities, for which different therapy should be appropriate [9].

In 2010, Chi et al., revealed that KIT-expressing interstitial cells of Cajal (ICC), that are presumed cells of origin of GIST, - also reveal high expression of the ETS transcription factor family member ETV1. The expression of ETV1 was found to be master regulator of an ICC-GIST specific transcription network that is further regulated by activated KIT and results in prolonged ETV1 protein stability and promotion of GIST tumorigenesis. However, the use of ETV1 as potential biomarker in GIST has to be confirmed [10]. In the recent work of Birner et al., ETV1 overexpression was not universally detected in GIST samples and clinical relevance was found to be low [11]. Moreover, the overexpression of MAPKAPK2, the inhibitor of ETV1 expression, was found to be an independent prognostic factor associated with significantly shorter disease-free survival of GIST patients [11].

In 2011, Delahaye et al., published their findings of the association between expression of specific isoform of natural killer cell receptor (NKp30c) and clinical outcome of GIST patients independent of their *KIT* mutational status. The relative overexpression of this immunosuppressive isoform identified GIST patients with unfavorable prognosis. Moreover in the study, the presence of specific SNP haplotype (including the NCR3*3790 SNP) was found to be associated with genetic control of NKp30 isoform expression pattern [12].

Some of the afore mentioned recently identified biomarkers can be utilized directly in future clinical trials that focus on the identification of novel targeted therapy agents for patients. Thus, the importance of identification of additional novel biomarkers lies not only in their potential utilization in disease diagnosis and prognosis specification and their potential to determinate patient subgroups with specific clinical phenotypes, but also in their usefulness in the design, setup and analysis of results of these clinical trials in retrospective as well as prospective manner. This can lead to identification of previously unknown associations between clinical phenotype and experimental therapy outcome.

2. Discovery of Novel Genes and Mutations Associated with Initiation and Progression of the Disease

In the era of genomic research, the simultaneous analysis of panels of genes, whole exomes or even genomes has led to the discovery of GIST associated gene mutations that occur with lower frequency. In 2013, Lawrence et al., studied the identification of novel genes associated with different types of tumors while analyzing more than three thousand tumor-normal pair samples. They developed and validated novel bioinformatic method for the detection of novel cancer related genes and showed that it can significantly shorten the list of candidate genes and lead to their faster and more effective validation [13]. In a recent study, performed on more than three thousand patient samples with 12 different tumor types, almost three hundred high-confidence cancer driver genes were identified, of which 165 were being discovered for the first time [14]. Later on in 2014, a large scale study, performed across 21 tumor types and on almost five thousand human cancer samples, revealed 33 novel genes that could be associated with carcinogenesis. Based on the saturation analysis, there are still many more mutated genes in clinically relevant frequencies that are waiting for discovery. Moreover in this study, it was suggested that the number of samples that should be analyzed on a genomic scale to identify these pools of genes was estimated to be 600 – 5000 for every cancer type [15]. In these studies, samples of patients with GIST were not analyzed. Therefore, further studies focusing on the discovery of novel genes responsible for the disease initiation or progression in GIST still need to be done in the future.

3. Novel Therapeutics Discovery and Utilization in GIST Treatment

Targeting KIT and PDGFRa receptor tyrosine kinases has led to the identification of imatinib (with different dosage of the drug for specific subgroups of patients) as a positive therapeutical answer for patients with GIST. Alternative TKI (i.e., sunitinib) is currently the "gold standard" therapy when standard dose of imatinib is not working as first line therapy or after secondary resistance to imatinib treatment occur. However, a significant proportion of GIST patients do not benefit from therapy with imatinib or sunitinib, become resistant while on treatment or develop severe adverse effects. In these situations, the two possible alternatives are ragorafenib and masitinib. Ragorafenib has showed its treatment efficacy [16] and is, as of February 2015, approved by the FDA for treatment of GIST patients who have experienced disease progression or developed intolerance while on previous imatinib or sunitinib therapy. On the other hand, masitinib is still in clinical trial phase. In the study of Adenis et al., masitinib revealed its potential to treat patients with advanced GIST after imatinib intolerance or failure and showed a therapeutical benefit comparable to sunitinib in these patients. Patients treated with masitinib experienced less toxicity than those receiving sunitinib, and had significantly lower occurrence of severe adverse events. Additionally, the median overall survival was significantly longer for patients receiving masitinib followed by post-progression addition of sunitinib when compared to patients treated directly with sunitinib in second-line therapy. The risk of progression while under treatment with masitinib was in the same range as for sunitinib [17].

In different subgroups of patients, especially those with "wild type" GIST, other TKI agents should be used. These therapies are based on targeting any of the downstream signaling cascade elements in which oncogenic mutation events have occurred. In 2013, the first report on successful treatment of patients, with "wild type" GIST and BRAF V600E mutation, with BRAF inhibitor dabrafenib, was published [18]. Based on recent identification of novel biomarkers associated with disease progression, novel targets for targeted therapy has recently been tested and are favorites for future studies. The IGF1R inhibitory effect of linsitinib will be studied in Phase 2 Study in Pediatric and Adult Wild Type Gastrointestinal Stromal Tumor patients (Clinical Trial Identifier NCT01560260). The potential of identification and clinical testing of ETV1 and MAPKAPK2 inhibitors for treatment of GIST patients was mentioned by previous studies [8, 9]. The ETV1 inhibitor represented by MEK162 showed, in experimental settings, increased tumor growth suppression in vitro and complete tumor regression in vivo using mouse models of Kit activation and ETV1 ablation [19]. Moreover, there is an ongoing phase 2 study for MEK 162 with the aim to test whether treatment with MEK162 demonstrates sufficient efficacy in select pathway-activated solid tumors (Clinical Trial Identifier NCT01885195).

4. Novel Approaches to Molecular Profiling of Tumor Tissue

Classical approaches to tumor tissue molecular analysis are based on biological samples gained with utilization of invasive methods represented by surgical tumor tissue removal or biopsy. Recently the possibility of detailed and comprehensive analysis of tumor DNA from patients' peripheral circulation was discovered based on analysis of circulating tumor DNA (ctDNA) gained by so called liquid biopsy. The possibility to scan cancer related changes in nonspecific (global hypomethylation and CNV analysis) as well as tumor type specific (tumor specific CNV and SNP analysis) manner brings novel dimension of cancer identification [20, 21]. Moreover, the digital nature of the currently available methods used for ctDNA analysis, represented mostly by massively parallel sequencing (MPS), allows quantitative analysis of molecular changes related to tumorigenesis. Together with the implementation of repeatedly performed liquid biopsies in different stages of the disease or times from beginning of therapy, it will be possible to monitor the mutation evolution of the tumor across time, and to quantify changes in tumor mass. Additionally, this method has enabled the study of tumor clonality and record intra-metastatic and inter-metastatic molecular heterogeneity that is typical for GIST. This allows detection and real time monitoring of newly emerging driver mutations or of mutations causing resistance to ongoing therapy and modification of the ongoing therapy in personalized manner [22]. A recent study focusing on targeted analysis of ctDNA samples in GIST patients has lead to the identification of significantly higher amounts of mutations - in ctDNA of patients with active disease compared to that in patients with complete remission. Therefore, the identification of tumor-specific mutations in the circulation of patients with GIST can be used as tumor-specific biomarker. The detection of resistance mutations might allow earlier treatment modification that obviates the need for repeated invasive tumor biopsies [23]. Moreover, based on optimistic results of pilot and validation studies performed on different types of cancers like the breast, ovarian, lung or colorectal cancer [22, 24-26], liquid biopsy genomic analysis based on MPS technology seems to be a promising tool in GIST management, offering a wide spectrum of research and clinical applications. Thus, the analysis of ctDNA in GIST patients can be used in variety of ways: as a basic tool for identification of novel biomarkers or therapy targets; as alternative source of tumor DNA overcoming the limitation of creating fresh tissue banks; to facilitate detailed molecular classification of the disease; and to define different molecular profiles of patients selected for clinical trials [27].

REFERENCES

[1] Casali PG. Successes and limitations of targeted cancer therapy in gastrointestinal stromal tumors. *Prog. Tumor Res.* 2014; 41:51-61.

[2] Sarlomo-Rikala M, Kovatich AJ, Barusevicius A, Miettinen M. CD117: a sensitive marker for gastrointestinal stromal tumors that is more specific than CD34. *Mod. Pathol.* 1998; 11(8):728-34.

[3] Heinrich MC, Corless CL, Duensing A et al., PDGFRA activating mutations in gastrointestinal stromal tumors. *Science* 2003; 299(5607):708-10.

[4] Hirota S, Isozaki K, Moriyama Y. Gain-of-function mutations of c-kit in human gastrointestinal stromal tumors. *Science* 1998; 279(5350):577-80.

[5] Joensuu H, Roberts PJ, Sarlomo-Rikala M et al., Effect of the tyrosine kinase inhibitor STI571 in a patient with a metastatic gastrointestinal stromal tumor. *N. Engl. J. Med.* 2001; 344(14):1052-6.

[6] Tornillo L. Gastrointestinal stromal tumor - an evolving concept. *Front Med.* (Lausanne) 2014; 1: 43.

[7] Miettinen M, Wang ZF, Lasota J. DOG1 antibody in the differential diagnosis of gastrointestinal stromal tumors: a study of 1840 cases. *Am. J. Surg. Pathol.* 2009; 33(9):1401-8.

[8] Doyle LA, Nelson D, Heinrich MC, Corless CL, Hornick JL. Loss of succinate dehydrogenase subunit B (SDHB) expression is limited to a distinctive subset of gastric wild-type gastrointestinal stromal tumours: a comprehensive genotype-phenotype correlation study. *Histopathology* 2012; 61(5):801-9.

[9] Beadling C, Patterson J, Justusson E, et al., Gene expression of the IGF pathway family distinguishes subsets of gastrointestinal stromal tumors wild type for KIT and PDGFRA. *Cancer Med.* 2013; 2(1):21-31.

[10] Chi P, Chen Y, Zhang L, et al., ETV1 is a lineage survival factor that cooperates with KIT in gastrointestinal stromal tumours. *Nature* 2010; 467(7317):849-53.

[11] Birner P, Beer A, Vinatzer U, et al., MAPKAP kinase 2 overexpression influences prognosis in gastrointestinal stromal tumors and associates with copy number variations on chromosome 1 and expression of p38 MAP kinase and ETV1. *Clin. Cancer Res.* 2012; 18(7):1879-87.

[12] Delahaye NF, Rusakiewicz S, Martins I, et al., Alternatively spliced NKp30 isoforms affect the prognosis of gastrointestinal stromal tumors. *Nat. Med.* 2011; 17(6):700-7.

[13] Lawrence MS, Stojanov P, Polak P, et al., Mutational heterogeneity in cancer and the search for new cancer-associated genes. *Nature* 2013; 499(7457):214-8.

[14] Tamborero D, Gonzalez-Perez A, Perez-Llamas C, et al., Comprehensive identification of mutational cancer driver genes across 12 tumor types. *Sci. Rep.* 2013; 3:2650.

[15] Lawrence MS, Stojanov P, Mermel CH, et al., Discovery and saturation analysis of cancer genes across 21 tumour types. *Nature* 2014; 505(7484):495-501.

[16] Demetri GD, Reichardt P, Kang YK, et al., Efficacy and safety of regorafenib for advanced gastrointestinal stromal tumours after failure of imatinib and sunitinib (GRID): an international, multicentre, randomised, placebo-controlled, phase 3 trial. *Lancet* 2013; 381(9863):295-302.

[17] Adenis A, Blay JY, Bui-Nguyen B, et al., Masitinib in advanced gastrointestinal stromal tumor (GIST) after failure of imatinib: a randomized controlled open-label trial. *Ann. Oncol.* 2014; 25(9):1762-9.

[18] Falchook GS, Trent JC, Heinrich MC, et al., BRAF mutant gastrointestinal stromal tumor: first report of regression with BRAF inhibitor dabrafenib (GSK2118436) and whole exomic sequencing for analysis of acquired resistance. *Oncotarget* 2013; 4(2):310-5.

[19] Ran L, Sirota I, Cao Z, et al., Combined inhibition of MAP kinase and KIT signaling synergistically destabilizes ETV1 and suppresses GIST tumor growth. *Cancer Discov.* 2015; 5(3):304-15.

[20] Chan KC, Jiang P, Chan CW, et al., Noninvasive detection of cancer-associated genome-wide hypomethylation and copy number aberrations by plasma DNA bisulfite sequencing. *Proc. Natl. Acad. Sci. USA* 2013; 110(47):18761-8.

[21] Chan KC, Jiang P, Zhang YW et al., Cancer genome scanning in plasma: detection of tumor-associated copy number aberrations, single-nucleotide variants, and tumoral heterogeneity by massively parallel sequencing. *Clin. Chem.* 2013; 59(1):211-24.

[22] Murtaza M, Dawson SJ, Tsui DW, et al., Non-invasive analysis of acquired resistance to cancer therapy by sequencing of plasma DNA. *Nature* 2013; 497(7447):108-12.

[23] Maier J, Lange T, Kerle I, et al., Detection of mutant free circulating tumor DNA in the plasma of patients with gastrointestinal stromal tumor harboring activating mutations of CKIT or PDGFRA. *Clin. Cancer Res.* 2013; 19(17):4854-67.

[24] Forshew T, Murtaza M, Parkinson C, et al., Noninvasive identification and monitoring of cancer mutations by targeted deep sequencing of plasma DNA. *Sci. Transl. Med.* 2012; 4(136):136ra68.

[25] Montagut C, Siravegna G, Bardelli A. Liquid biopsies to evaluate early therapeutic response in colorectal cancer. *Ann. Oncol.* 2015 [pii: mdv228]

[26] Rothe F, Laes JF, Lambrechts D, et al., Plasma circulating tumor DNA as an alternative to metastatic biopsies for mutational analysis in breast cancer. *Ann. Oncol.* 2014; 25(10):1959-65.

[27] Nannini M, Astolfi A, Urbini M, Biasco G, Pantaleo MA. Liquid biopsy in gastrointestinal stromal tumors: a novel approach. *J. Transl. Med.* 2014; 12:210.

In: Gastrointestinal Stromal Tumors in Adults … ISBN: 978-1-63483-679-1
Editor: Atif A. Ahmed

Chapter 9

MANAGEMENT OF GASTROINTESTINAL STROMAL TUMORS: PRESENT AND FUTURE DIRECTIONS

***Gloria Ravegnini*[*] *and Sabrina Angelini*[†]**
Pharmacogenetic and Pharmacogenomic Unit,
University of Bologna, Bologna, Italy

ABSTRACT

Gastrointestinal stromal tumors (GIST) are the most common tumors of the gastrointestinal tract. They are characterized by gain of function mutations in KIT or PDGFRA genes. Imatinib is the gold standard therapy for the management of these tumors and it led a terrific improvement in GIST patients' prognosis. GIST patients respond very well to the tyrosine kinase inhibitor (TKI) imatinib for about 18-36 months; however, the occurrence of resistance after this time is extremely common. Clearly, TKIs have been developed as target therapy for GIST with specific mutations in KIT and PDGFRA. Unfortunately, 10-15% of all GIST are classified as wild-type (WT) GIST, not harboring any mutation in KIT/PDGFRA. This subgroup of patients, although characterized by a unique phenotype, are however treated with TKI. Despite all these observations, imatinib remains the only first choice and the best treatment in GIST patients

[*] Email: gloria.ravegnini2@unibo.it.
[†] Email: s.angelini@unibo.it.

In view of these considerations, the identification of new molecules, beyond TKIs is highly needed. The aim of this chapter is to highlight the state of the art of GIST management, with particular focus on TKIs resistant patients and wild-type GIST.

INTRODUCTION

Imatinib had radically changed the history of gastrointestinal stromal tumor (GIST) management and prognosis. Starting from its approval in 2000, the prognosis for patients with unresectable disease has dramatically changed from a median overall survival of 12 months to a survival approaching 5 years or more. Usually, GIST patients respond very well to the tyrosine kinase inhibitor (TKI) imatinib for about 18-36 months; however, the occurrence of resistance after this time is extremely common [1, 2]. For patients with GIST who develop disease progression during imatinib treatment or are intolerant to imatinib, sunitinib and regorafenib, second and third generation TKIs respectively, represent the standard therapy [3, 4].

Imatinib mesylate (GLEEVEC® formerly STI571, developed by Novartis Pharma AG, Basel, Switzerland) is a TKI acting against several different tyrosine kinases, including ABL, BCR-ABL, KIT, PDGFRA, PDGFRB and CSF1R. Its structure mimics adenosine triphosphate (ATP) and binds competitively to the ATP binding site of the targeted kinases. This prevents substrate phosphorylation and the resulting signaling, thereby inhibiting proliferation and survival [5, 6]. Sunitinib malate (SUTENT®, formerly SU11248, developed by Pfizer, New York, USA) is an orally administered multitarget receptor TKI, which acts on TK, including KIT, PDGFR (α and β), VEGFR (1, 2, and 3), FLT3, CSF-1R, and RET; additionally it has demonstrated remarkable anti-angiogenic properties. Sunitinib, similar to imatinib, inhibits the ATP binding site, but has demonstrated to be active in imatinib-resistant GIST [7]. Regorafenib (STIVARGA, formerly BAY 73-4506, developed by BAYER, Levurkusen, Germany) is an orally available multikinase inhibitor with activity against multiple targets, including KIT, PDGFR, VEGFR (1, 2, and 3), TIE2, RET, FGFR 1, RAF, and p38 mitogen-activated protein kinase (MAPK) [8].

Clearly, all these three TKIs have been developed as target therapy for GIST with specific mutations in KIT and PDGFRA, characterizing about 75-85% of GISTs. Unfortunately, 10-15% of all GIST are classified as wild-type (WT) GIST, not harboring any known activating mutation in KIT/PDGFRA.

This subgroup of patients, although characterized by a unique phenotype, are however treated with TKI. This undoubtedly highlights the lack of alternative treatments for WT GISTs. This lack of alternative treatments also reflects on patients harboring the PDGFRA D842V mutation, which are known to be totally resistant to imatinib. Furthermore, there is a growing body of evidence of inter-patient variability in imatinib response, due to the presence of genetic polymorphisms in imatinib related metabolizing and transporter coding enzymes and in folate-related genes [9-12]. Despite all these observations, imatinib remains the only first choice and the best treatment in GIST patients. Second- and third-line TKIs have only limited clinical efficacy, probably as a result of imatinib-resistant mutation heterogeneity, and patients with advanced GIST eventually die of the disease [13-15]. In view of these considerations imatinib resistance remains the greatest challenge in the management of GISTs.

AN UPDATE ON THE TYROSIN KINASE INHIBITORS ALTERNATIVES

To date, based on the molecular mechanism of action, there are mainly five groups of drugs, offering an attractive alternative to imatinib:

- PI3K/AKT/mTOR Pathway Inhibitors
- Heat Shock Protein 90 Inhibitors
- Insulin Growth Factor Receptor Inhibitors
- Monoclonal antibodies
- VEGFR inhibitors

Table 1. Summarizing the main molecules in trial for the GIST treatment

PI3K/AKT/mTOR inhibitor	HSP90 inhibitors	IGFR1 inhibitors	Monoclonal AB	VEGFR inhibitors
BKM120	IPI-504	R1507	Ipilimumab	Cederanib
GDC-0941	IPI-493	Linsitinib	Olaratumab	
SF1126	STA-9090			
BEZ235	BIIB021			
BYL719	AT13387			
GDC-0980	AUY922			
Everolimus				
Sirolimus				

PI3K/AKT/mTOR Pathway Inhibitors

PI3K/AKT/mTOR hyperactivation pathway is the result of KIT/PDGFRA receptor activation in GIST and is common in both mutant and WT GIST [14, 16]. In imatinib resistant GIST, this pathway is even more activated than imatinib sensitive. In this view, the inhibition of PI3K/AKT/mTOR path could be a strong and rational therapeutic approach.

Basically, these inhibitors act specifically against one the main actors of this pathway: mTOR, PI3K or AKT. mTOR pathway, and mTOR in particular, has attracted the research interest, as it is an intracellular protein kinase promoting cancer cell growth and survival, and it clearly contributes to the pathgenesis of a variety of malignancies [17].

Different trials focused specifically on mTOR inhibitors as rapamycin (also known as rypamicin) analogs or everolimus in combination with imatinib. Rapamycin acts also as inducer of authophagy, reducing the expression of both phospho- and total KIT, which leads to enhanced apoptosis of KIT-expressing cells [18]. Overall mTOR inhibition associated with autophagy induction might represent a potential therapeutic strategy for TKI-refractory GIST. Another promising approach, which warranted further investigation, is the combination everolimus and imatinib. A phase I-II study has shown an improvement in median progression free survival in GIST patients with progressive disease on imatinib and sunitinib [17].

Another interesting option is represented by mTOR upstream target genes, such as PI3K or AKT; indeed, it is conceivable that, blocking these protein activities, the final effect would be more effective. A preclinical study by Bauer et al., have corroborated this hypothesis, showing that the PI3K/AKT pathway is a therapeutic target, particularly relevant in imatinib-resistant GIST, even in the absence of KIT expression [19]. To date, BKM120 and BYL 719 in combination with imatinib are under phase I clinical trial as a third line treatment option, for GIST patients with progressive disease after imatinib and sunitinib.

Heat Shock Protein 90 Inhibitors

Heat shock proteins (Hsp) are highly conserved proteins, working as a molecular chaperon for several cellular proteins, and essential for normal cell viability and growth. Hsp90, in particular, interacts with proteins and mediates cell signaling involved in essential processes such as proliferation, cell cycle control, angiogenesis and apoptosis. It is involved in different oncogenic processes and for this reason its inhibition could represent a reasonable anticancer strategy [20]. KIT/PDGFRA are Hsp90 clients to stabilize their folding and this leads Hsp90 inhibitors to be excellent candidates to overpass the TKI resistance in GIST [21, 22]. Previous studies in cell lines and *in vivo* models have confirmed HSP90 inhibition might be an effective treatment option for GIST [23-28]. Hsp90 inhibition involves competitive binding to its N-terminal ATP binding pocket, which prevents the ATPase activity responsible for stabilization of client proteins [22]. One of the first Hsp90 inhibitors developed was the 17-Allylamino-17- demethoxygeldanamycin (17-AGG); it was tested, with interesting findings, by Bauer et al., in both imatinib-sensitive and imatinib-resistant GIST cell lines. The first results showed that 17-AGG had an effect in GIST cell lines KIT positive as a result of KIT oncoprotein inhibition [23]. This initial finding showed Hsp90 inhibition might represent a promising strategy to overcome imatinib resistance in GIST. The main issue of 17-AGG therapeutic strategy was related to the hepatotoxicity (due to bioreduction by NQO1 to the toxic DT-diaphorase) which greatly limits the use [22-24]. In light of this toxicity, new compounds, Hsp90 inhibitors, have been developed, including IPI-493, IPI-504, STA-9090, BIIB021, AT13387, and AUY922. All these molecules have demonstrated, in both imatinib sensitive and imatinib resistant GIST cell lines, cell grown inhibition with the abolishment of KIT activity and KIT downstream cascade [25-29]. To date, STA-9090, BIIB021 and AUY922 are the most promising agents, and are in a phase II clinical trial showing promising results in imatinib and sunitinib resistant GIST [14].

Insulin Growth Factor Receptor Inhibitors

Insulin-like growth factor (IGF) cascade pathway plays a critical role in the growth and development of many tissues and regulates overall cell growth. The IGF system is composed of the IGF ligands (IGF-1 and IGF-2), receptors (IGFR) [30, 31] and its activation leads to activation of the mitogen-activated protein kinase (MAPK) and PI3K cascades [28]. Over-expression of IGFR1 has been characterized in many cancer types and it has been proposed a target for anticancer molecules [31]. In particular, IGFR1 overexpression characterizes WT GIST and pediatric GIST [32], whereas no activation have been observed in KIT/PFGFRα mutant GISTs [33]. In view of this consideration

IGFR1 represents an interesting target for this subgroup of patients, still orphans of a specific treatment.

Despite the interest about IGFR1 inhibitors, to date, there are only two of these inhibitors in trials for GIST patients, Linsitinib and R1507. Linsitinib (formerly known as OSI-906, developed by OSI Pharmaceuticals) is an oral inhibitor of both IGF1R and the insulin receptor (IR). A phase II trial is ongoing to evaluate Linsitinib in pediatric and adult patients with WT GIST [34, 35]. R1507 is a fully human IGF-1R monoclonal antibody in phase Ib trial, used for different refractory advanced solid malignancies, and its use has demonstrated promising results. With regard to GIST patients, R1507 has been used as compassionate drug in a young woman but, at the moment, R1507 is no longer under development [34].

Monoclonal Antibodies

Immune surveillance presumes that pre-malignant lesion or early tumor cells can be killed or at least controlled by specific cells of the immune system. Unfortunately, advanced tumors develop the ability to evade immune control and as a consequence, the majority of the advanced cancers are poorly immunogenic.

Immunotherapy aims to recover patient´s inefficient or suppressed immunity, leading to sustained cytolytic attacks against tumor cells, which would ideally result in the eradication of cancer [36]. In light of this, monoclonal antibodies (Mabs) might play an important role among the innovative immunotherapy approaches. To date, two Mabs are under evaluation in clinical trial for GIST treatment. A phase I study is employing the combination of ipilimumab and dasatinib in patients with unresectable or metastatic GIST. The main goal is to assess the safety and tolerability of treatment with ipilimumab in combination with dasatinib in subjects with GIST and other advanced sarcomas [37].

The other Mab in clinical trial is Olaratumab, a Mab for PDGFRA that selectively binds to PDGFRA, blocking the binding of its ligand, PDGF. A phase II study has evaluated the tumor response previously treated patients with unresectable/metastatic GIST however, to date, no results have been released [38].

VEGFR Inhibitors

Usually, the tumors arise due to loss of control of cell proliferation, however when the tumor reaches a size of 1–2 mm, it has to gain angiogenic properties to counteract the onset of necrosis. For this reason, the cancer begins to express several pro-angiogenic factors, as vascular endothelial growth factor (VEGF) and thereby the equilibrium between pro- and anti-angiogenic substances changes [39, 40].

The smaller GIST have a size <2cm but they can reach 10 cm or more and it has been seen VEGF plays an important role in GIST growth and metastasis [40]

Cediranib is a potent VEGF inhibitor with activity against VEGF receptors 1, 2 and 3 and KIT. This VEGF inhibitor is in a phase II study evaluating its antitumor activity in patients with metastatic GIST resistant/ intolerant to imatinib, or metastatic soft-tissue sarcomas [40]. To determine the antitumor activity of cediranib, changes in 2[18F]fluoro-2-deoxy-Dglucose positron emission tomography (18FDG-PET) has used. Unfortunately, only 40% of patients showed disease stabilization for more than 16 weeks with a median progression free survival of 2 months [41, 42].

Repurposing of Small Molecule Therapeutics

Recently, Passetto et al, evaluated a large library of FDA-approved drugs regardless the therapeutic indications. They identified eight molecules - auranofin, bortezomib, carbimazole, digoxin, gentian violet, idarubicin, ouabain, and fludarabine phosphate (F-AMP)- showing synergy with and/or overcame resistance to imatinib in GIST cell lines (GIST-T1, GIST882, GIST-T1-10R). In particular, among these, F-AMP seems to be the most promising since it induces cytotoxicity in GIST cells, including in the imatinib resistant one. F-AMP in combination with imatinib showed greater inhibition of GIST cell proliferation when compared with the single treatment alone. The success of the combination imatinib-F-AMP has been also confirmed in *in vivo* experiments. This results identified F-AMP as a promising therapy for the treatment of GISTs, with the potential to be administered in combination with imatinib or for treatment of imatinib–refractory tumors [43].

TOWARD NEW HORIZONS

Next-Generation Sequencing (NGS) and Personalized Therapy

Besides the approved drugs and the new molecules in trials, research is focusing on different fields with promising results.

Indeed, because GIST is a very heterogeneous group of patients and the resistance mechanisms can be very various as well, it is challenging to develop next-generation therapies that can address the majority of, if not all, resistance mechanisms. High-throughput screening techniques have led to identifying novel relevant genes in GIST. Recently, Schoppmann et al., identified 10 target genes in GIST using a novel approach combining DNA arrays, exome sequencing, and immunohistochemistry [44]. These candidate genes could have pathogenic and prognostic significance in GIST. In particular the data indicated an important involvement of the MAP kinase pathway in GIST, suggesting that the inclusion of MAP kinase pathway parameters in future clinical studies might be of potential benefit for the patients.

These sensitive techniques allow to get a clear picture of the tumor alterations pattern, which can even vary between different progressing metastases in each patient. Performing a whole genome analysis using a massively parallel sequencing approach Nannini and collaborators analyzed 16 GIST samples included WT-KIT, WT-PDGFRA, WT-SDH, and WT-RAS cases. Interestingly, they found that quadruple-WT GIST had an own expression signature, distinct from SDH-mutant GIST as well as KIT/PDGFR mutant GIST [45]. The finding is important because drives the rationale for which this group is unique and separated from other GIST, and clinicians should take it into account this difference in choosing the best drug for a given patient.

Beyond the specific mutations of the tumor, the germline genome could play an important role in the final clinical outcome as well. In light of this, is important considering the pharmacogenetic variants that could impact the drug metabolism and transport. Indeed, it is well known that any drug, starting from its intake, undergoes a specific pharmacokinetics itinerary, and certainly this itinerary has a role in drug efficacy and side effects [46]. As reported by few studies, some genetic polymorphisms could impact the therapeutic response to imatinib in GIST. Indeed, it seems that polymorphisms in transporter genes, for instance OCTN1, OCTN2 or ABCG2, might have an influence in imatinib response [9, 10, 12]. On the same way, genome-wide pharmacogenetic studies, in particular the Drug Metabolizing Enzymes and Transporters (DMET) array, may represent a novel approach for the identification of markers of imatinib response and toxicity [47]. Indeed the DMET platform permits to genotype simultaneously a set of 1936 variants in 225 genes involved in drug absorption, distribution, metabolism and elimination (ADME), representing a useful way to scan the genome for associations between variations in the ADME, the pharmacodynamic and outcomes of drug treatment [47].

A growing body of literature regarding the issue of personalized medicine is represented by microRNA (miRNA) deregulation. miRNA are a class of short noncoding RNAs, playing a relevant role in several biological processes, such as differentiation, proliferation and apoptosis [48]. MiRNA deregulation is emerging as having a relevant role in GIST biology, including disease development and progression, clinical outcome and drug resistance. Many studies have been conducted in the last years, however the major concern is the small consensus among the deregulated miRNA signature between the different studies [48]. Nonetheless, the majority of them agree to emphasize the importance of miR-221 and 222, which have been reported by four different groups as implicated in KIT expression regulation [49-52]. Specifically, miR-221 and -222 overexpression regulate the TK expression level in a negative manner and, as a result, these two miRNA could be important therapeutic targets for the GIST management.

REFERENCES

[1] Balachandran VP, DeMatteo RP. Gastrointestinal stromal tumors: who should get imatinib and for how long? *Adv Surg* 2014; 48:165-83.

[2] Nishida T, Doi T, Naito Y. Tyrosine kinase inhibitors in the treatment of unresectable or metastatic gastrointestinal stromal tumors. *Expert Opin Pharmacother*. 2014; 15(14):1979-89.

[3] Songdej N, von Mehren M. GIST treatment options after tyrosine kinase inhibitors. *Curr Treat Options Oncol* 2014; 15(3):493-506.

[4] Ferraro D, Zalcberg J. Regorafenib in gastrointestinal stromal tumors: clinical evidence and place in therapy. *Ther Adv Med Oncol.* 2014; 6(5):222-8.

[5] Pidhorecky I, Cheney RT, Kraybill W et al. Gastrointestinal stromal tumors: current diagnosis, biologic behavior, and management. *Ann Surg Oncol. 2000*; 7(9):705-12.

[6] Beham AW, Schaefer IM, Schüler P, et al. Gastrointestinal stromal tumors. *Int J Colorectal Dis.* 2012; 27(6):689-700.

[7] Demetri GD, Heinrich MC, Fletcher JA, et al. Molecular target modulation, imaging, and clinical evaluation of gastrointestinal stromal tumor patients treated with sunitinib malate after imatinib failure. *Clin Cancer Res.* 2009; 15(18):5902-9.

[8] Demetri GD, Reichardt P, Kang YK, et al. Efficacy and safety of regorafenib for advanced gastrointestinal stromal tumours after failure of imatinib and sunitinib (GRID): an international, multicentre, randomised, placebo-controlled, phase 3 trial. *Lancet* 2013; 381(9863):295-302.

[9] Angelini S, Pantaleo MA, Ravegnini G et al. Polymorphisms in OCTN1 and OCTN2 transporters genes are associated with prolonged time to progression in unresectable gastrointestinal stromal tumours treated with imatinib therapy. *Pharmacol Res* 2013; 68(1):1-6.

[10] Angelini S, Ravegnini G, Nannini M, et al. Folate-related polymorphisms in gastrointestinal stromal tumours: susceptibility and correlation with tumour characteristics and clinical outcome. *Eur J Hum Genet.* 2015; 23(6):817-23.

[11] Angelini S, Ravegnini G, Fletcher JA, et al. Clinical relevance of pharmacogenetics in gastrointestinal stromal tumor treatment in the era of personalized therapy *Pharmacogenomics.* 2013; 14(8):941-56.

[12] Koo DH, Ryu MH, Ryoo BY, et al. Association of ABCG2 polymorphism with clinical efficacy of imatinib in patients with gastrointestinal stromal tumor. *Cancer Chemother Pharmacol.* 2015; 75(1):173-82.

[13] Ran L, Sirota I, Cao Z, et al. Combined inhibition of MAP kinase and KIT signaling synergistically destabilizes ETV1 and suppresses GIST tumor growth. *Cancer Discov.* 2015; 5(3):304-15.

[14] Songdej N, von Mehren M. GIST treatment options after tyrosine kinase inhibitors. *Curr Treat Options Oncol.* 2014; 15(3):493-506.

[15] Heinrich MC, Corless CL, Blanke CD, et al. (2006). Molecular correlates of imatinib resistance in gastrointestinal stromal tumors. *J Clin Oncol* 2006; 24: 4764–4774.

[16] Patel S. Exploring novel therapeutic targets in GIST: focus on the PI3K/Akt/mTOR pathway. *Curr Oncol Rep.* 2013; 15(4):386-95.

[17] Schöffski P, Reichardt P, Blay J-Y, et al. A phase I-II study of everolimus (RAD001) in combination with imatinib in patients with imatinib-resistant gastrointestinal stromal tumors. *Ann Oncol* 2010; 21(10):1990–8.

[18] Hsueh YS, Chang HH, Chiang NJ, Yen CC, Li CF, Chen LT MTOR inhibition enhances NVP-AUY922-induced autophagy-mediated KIT degradation and cytotoxicity in imatinib-resistant gastrointestinal stromal tumors. *Oncotarget* 2014; 5(22):11723-36.

[19] Bauer S, Duensing A, Demetri GD et al. KIT oncogenic signaling mechanisms in imatinib-resistant gastrointestinal stromal tumor: PI3-kinase/AKT is a crucial survival pathway. *Oncogene* 2007; 26(54): 7560–8.

[20] Sankhala KK, Mita MM, Mita AC, Takimoto CH. Heat shock proteins: a potential anticancer target. *Curr Drug Targets.* 2011; 12(14):2001-8.

[21] Smyth T, Van Looy T, Curry JE, et al. The HSP90 inhibitor, AT13387, is effective against imatinib-sensitive and -resistant gastrointestinal stromal tumor models. *Mol Cancer Ther* 2012; 11(8):1799-808.

[22] Trepel J, Mollapour M, Giaccone G. Targeting the dynamic HSP90 complex in cancer. *Nat Rev Cancer* 2010; 10(8):537–49.

[23] Bauer S, Yu LK, Demetri GD, Fletcher JA. Heat shock protein 90 inhibition in imatinib-resistant gastrointestinal stromal tumor. *Cancer Res* 2006; 66(18):9153-61.

[24] Fumo G, Akin C, Metcalfe DD, et al. 17- Allylamino-17-demethoxygeldanamycin (17-AAG) is effective in down-regulating mutated, constitutively activated KIT protein in human mast cells. *Blood.* 2004; 103(3):1078–84.

[25] Fletcher JA, Debiec-Rychter M, Swank S, et al. HSP90 inhibitor STA-9090 potently suppresses secondary KIT kinase-domain mutations responsible for gastrointestinal stromal tumor (GIST) progression during imatinib therapy. *Mol Cancer Ther* 2009;8 Suppl 1:B184.

[26] Floris G, Debiec-Rychter M, Wozniak A, et al. The heat shock protein 90 inhibitor IPI-504 induces KIT degradation, tumor shrinkage, and cell proliferation arrest in xenograft models of gastrointestinal stromal tumors. *Mol Cancer Ther* 2011;10(10):1897–908.

[27] Floris G, Sciot R, Wozniak A, et al. The Novel HSP90 inhibitor, IPI-493, is highly effective in human gastrostrointestinal stromal tumor xenografts carrying heterogeneous KIT mutations. *Clin Cancer Res* 2011; 17(17):5604–14.

[28] Dewaele B, Wasag B, Cools J, et al. Activity of dasatinib, a dual SRC/ABL kinase inhibitor, and IPI-504, a heat shock protein 90 inhibitor, against gastrointestinal stromal tumor-associated PDGFR AD842V mutation. *Clin Cancer Res* 2008; 14:5749–58.

[29] Smyth T, Van Looy T, Curry JE, et al. The HSP90 inhibitor, AT13387, is effective against imatinib-sensitive and -resistant gastrointestinal stromal tumor models. *Mol Cancer Ther* 2012; 11(8):1799–808.

[30] LeRoith D, Roberts CT. The insulin-like growth factor system and cancer. *Cancer Lett* 2003; 195:127–137.

[31] Tarn C, Rink L, Merkel E, et al. Insulin-like growth factor 1 receptor is a potential therapeutic target for gastrointestinal stromal tumors. *Proc Natl Acad Sci U S A*. 2008; 105(24):8387-92.

[32] Belinsky MG, Rink L, Flieder DB, et al. Overexpression of insulin-like growth factor 1 receptor and frequent mutational inactivation of SDHA in wild-type SDHB-negative gastrointestinal stromal tumors. *Genes Chromosomes Cancer*. 2013; 52(2):214-24.

[33] Tarn C, Rink L, Merkel E, et al. Insulin-like growth factor 1 receptor is a potential therapeutic target for gastrointestinal stromal tumors. *Proc Natl Acad Sci USA*. 2008; 105(24):8387–92.

[34] Saponara M, Pantaleo MA, Nannini M, et al. Treatments for gastrointestinal stromal tumors that are resistant to standard therapies. *Future Oncol* 2014; 10(13):2045-59.

[35] https://www.clinicaltrials.gov/ct2/show/NCT01560260.

[36] Jr PK, Otahal P, Klener P. Principles of Cancer Immunotherapy. Curr Pharm Biotechnol. 2015. [Epub ahead of print]

[37] https://www.clinicaltrials.gov/ct2/show/record/NCT01643278.

[38] https://clinicaltrials.gov/ct2/show/record/NCT01316263.

[39] Versleijen-Jonkers YM, Vlenterie M, van de Luijtgaarden AC, et al. Anti-angiogenic therapy, a new player in the field of sarcoma treatment. *Crit Rev Oncol Hematol* 2014; 91(2):172-85.

[40] Alturkmani HJ, Pessetto ZY, Godwin AK. Beyond standard therapy: drugs under investigation for the treatment of gastrointestinal stromal tumor. *Expert Opin Investig Drugs* 2015; 24(8):1045-58.

[41] Judson I, Scurr M, Gardner K et al. Phase II study of cediranib in patients with advanced gastrointestinal stromal tumors or soft-tissue sarcoma. *Clin Cancer Res* 2014; 20(13):3603-12.

[42] https://clinicaltrials.gov/show/NCT00385203

[43] Pessetto ZY, Ma Y, Hirst JJ, et al. Drug repurposing identifies a synergistic combination therapy with imatinib mesylate for gastro-intestinal stromal tumor. *Mol Cancer Ther* 2014; 13(10):2276-87.

[44] Schoppmann SF, Vinatzer U, Popitsch N, et al. Novel clinically relevant genes in gastrointestinal stromal tumors identified by exome sequencing. *Clin Cancer Res*. 2013; 19(19):5329-39.

[45] Nannini M, Astolfi A, Urbini M, et al. Integrated genomic study of quadruple-WT GIST (KIT/PDGFRA/SDH/RAS pathway wild-type GIST). *BMC Cancer.* 2014; 14:685.

[46] Ravegnini G, Nannini M, Sammarini G e al. Personalized Medicine in Gastrointestinal Stromal Tumor (GIST): Clinical Implications of the Somatic and Germline DNA Analysis. *Int J Mol Sci 2015;* 16(7):15592-608.

[47] Sissung T, English B, Venzon D, et al. Clinical pharmacology and pharmacogenetics in a genomics era: The DMET platform. *Pharmacogenomics.* 2010; 11(1):89-103.

[48] Nannini M, Ravegnini G, Angelini S, et al. MicroRNAs profiling in gastrointestinal tumors: implication as diagnostic and prognostic markers. *Epigenomics* 2015 [in press].

[49] Gits C, van Kuijk P.; Jonkers M, et al. MiR-17-92 and miR-221/222 cluster members target KIT and ETV1 in human gastrointestinal stromal tumours. *Br J Cancer* 2013; 109:1625-1635.

[50] Haller F, von Heydebreck A, Zhang, J, et al. Localization- and mutation-dependent microRNA (miRNA) expression signatures in gastrointestinal stromal tumours (GISTs), with a cluster of co-expressed miRNAs located at 14q32.31. *J Pathol* 2010; 220:71-86.

[51] Koelz M, Lense J, Wrba F, et al. Down-regulation of miR-221 and miR-222 correlates with pronounced KIT expression in gastrointestinal stromal tumors. *Int J Oncol* 2011; 38:503-511.

[52] Subramanian S, Lui W, Lee C, et al. MicroRNA expression signature of human sarcomas. *Oncogene* 2008; 27:2015-2026.

INDEX

B

C

D

E

H

I

J

K

L

M

N

O

P

Q

R

S

X

Y